EAT MORE TO LOSE MORE
Diet Book

BY NUTRITION EXPERT
UNNI GREENE

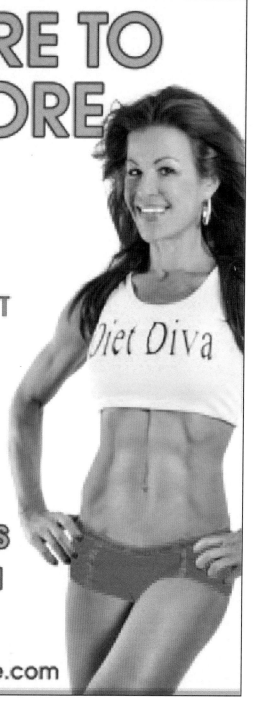

THE DIET DIVA REVEALS HER TOP NUTRIONAL SECRETS TO SLIMMING DOWN BY EATING MORE!

www.EatMoreToLoseMore.com

ISBN: 0615740308
ISBN-13: 9780615740300

MEDICAL DISCLAIMER

The information is this work is in no way intended as medical advice or as a substitute for medical counseling. This publication contains the opinions and ideas of its author. It is intended to provide helpful and informative material on the subjects addressed in the publication. It is sold with the understanding that the author and publisher are not engaged in rendering medical, health, psychological, or any other kind of personal professional services in the book. If the reader requires personal medical, health, or other assistance or advice, a competent professional should be consulted. The author and publisher specifically disclaim all responsibility for any liability or loss, personal or otherwise, that is incurred as a consequence, directly or indirectly, of the use and application of the contents of this book..

Table of Contents

Acknowledgments

This book is dedicated to my wonderful family, who watched patiently as I labored for endless hours over this book. They always believe in me, and they encourage me to reach higher and try harder: my incredible children Erica, Alana, Matthew, and Marcus, and my steadfast partner, William. Without them, I could not have achieved this.

This book is also dedicated to my dear friend Jennifer Nicole Lee who has given me her guidance, support, and endless enthusiasm. Without her, none of this would be possible.

I also dedicate this book to my clients, for inspiring me to reach higher and do better every day so that I can help them be the best they can be.

I also dedicate this book to *you* reading this book right now: it is my hope that with the help of this book, you, too, can experience the joy of being as fit and healthy as you can be and enjoy all aspects of your life at your physical peak by learning to eat more to lose more.

Thank you,

Unni Greene

The Diet Diva

Foreword by Jennifer Nicole Lee

When Unni "The Diet Diva" Greene asked me to write the foreword to her book, I was honored. I jumped at the opportunity, as I finally got to return the favor of her writing the foreword to my Fun Fit Foodie Cookbook. She is an angel to many, including me!

I have to say it's absolutely mind-boggling that Unni is only a few years away from turning fifty with four kids, yet she has been able to defy the "norm" by having a rock-hard, super-fit, tight and toned body—with boundless energy! What are her secrets? Well, all of her nutritional secrets are revealed in this very book you are about to read! Get ready to re-ignite your passion for food, redefine what you think eating healthy is all about, and embrace the new nutritional journey that "The Diet Diva" is about to take you on. Buckle your seatbelts and get ready for a healthy, happy ride!

With her years of expertise, her endless client list, and her sincere dedication to and focus on her passion, Unni is not only talking the talk but also walking the walk! This is what I adore about her. She is not "preaching from a pulpit" but speaks to you "sister to sister," like a near-and-dear friend! And when you read this book, you will see and feel her passion for nutrition and helping others achieve their nutritional goals. She loves what she does, and it shows. Luckily we are all here to reap the benefits of this super-passionate specialist in sports nutrition and supplementation.

Having been in the fitness industry for close to a decade, I have had the advantage of meeting all of the "best of the best" in fitness, sports and nutrition. However, hands down, Unni "The Diet Diva" Greene is in a league of her own, and really stands apart from the sea of "so-called" experts. She has earned her stripes in making sure her entire family and her clients all eat optimally—while taking care of her own dietary needs as well!

As many of you know, I use the world "believe" a lot in my keynote speeches, books, and personal and business branding. It's a strong message that I rely upon to evoke a notion that all things are possible. I believe in Unni, and her messages—and soon you will, too. You will see for yourself your own personal "miracles" that you will enjoy by simply believing in her "Eat More to Lose More" principles! I believe in Unni, as she practices what she preaches, and we can all see it works!

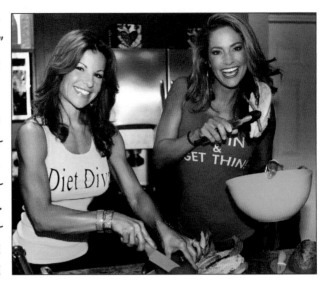

Also, there is a huge element of trust in Unni's expertise. Unni has worked with me on many fitness projects, productions, book signings, and keynote speeches, and her vast expertise, knowledge, and professionalism always shines through. She takes her passion for nutrition seriously, making sure you will learn so much, thus empowering you to truly connect with what you are putting into your body.

Please note that Unni has worked tremendously hard on creating this e-book for you to enjoy. She has put her heart and soul (and favorite recipes) into this "treasure trove" of dietary delights! Again, wearing as many hats as Unni does, time is not a luxury for this super-busy and in-demand fitness expert. Every year she is an executive expert at my annual JNL World Conference, giving keynote speeches to the most powerful, prolific, and passionate fitness, wellness, and nutritional enthusiasts from around the globe. She is also the owner of the private training facility SoMi Fitness. So as you can see, she has gone way beyond to give you her very best tips to help you get trim and slim—all by eating more! No deprivation! Now that's the part that I *love*!

Jennifer Nicole Lee

"The Fun Fit Foodie" www.JenniferNicoleLee.com

Part I

Get Started on Your New Path to Health

I wrote this book for *you*. It will explain the basics of how your metabolism works and how it everything that you put into your body affects it. I will also explain why you have to eat more to lose more. Who am I, you wonder? I am a certified personal master trainer and a sports nutrition specialist. I have a bachelor's degree from the University of Miami, and I have many certifications in different fitness and nutrition specialties. I am also a health and wellness expert and celebrity coach. I hold certifications in training and nutrition from ISSA, NFPT 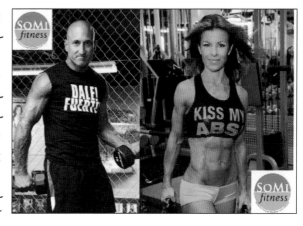 and NASM. I train and counsel countless professional athletes, mothers, fathers, teenagers, fitness models—you name it. It is my passion and pleasure to share my knowledge of health, fitness, and nutrition with others, so that they, too, may be able to reach their physical peak and optimal health.

In addition to being a health, fitness, and nutrition expert, I am the very proud mother of four beautiful children. If you are also a mom, you know all the challenges and rewards that brings. Additionally, I am the co-owner of a private training facility in South Miami called SoMi Fitness with my partner in the gym as well as in life, William Del Sol.

Although I have lived in the United States for the past thirty years, I actually grew up in Sweden. A very active child, I spent my childhood and adolescence as a semi-professional figure skater. Growing up with the required discipline for succeeding in sports and in a family that was very health conscious, I developed a love for all things fitness and nutrition from a very early age. As a young athlete, I learned that what I put into my body and how I trained it really affected my performance. I had to train a minimum of three hours per day and learned early on how to eat healthy to stay competitive.

When I was seventeen years old, I moved to Miami to attend the University of Miami. Throughout college, I earned some money by working part time as an aerobics' instructor at Lady of America. My love for fitness was growing strong, and in my free time I enjoyed running, swimming, and other water sports as well. I studied and graduated with a bachelor's degree in business administration and finance. I loved living in Miami, with its multicultural way of life, its endless sunshine and the many opportunities that I encountered. I decided to make Miami my home.

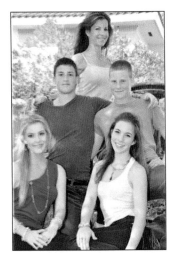

I got married and started my family in my early twenties. Being a very busy mom of four small children left very little time for me to take care of my own health and fitness needs. I was constantly taking care of others and putting myself and my own needs last. Through the years, I have shared many of the same struggles that you have. Although I was never clinically overweight, there were times when my workouts were nonexistent and my nutrition was very poor. I have been pregnant and given birth four times, with all the weight struggles and body transformations that go along with that.

I raised my four children and worked in business for many years. While I thoroughly enjoyed this, I had very little time leftover for myself. For many years, the only exercise I had time to do was to get up at five in the morning to squeeze in a quick run before the kids got up. Sometimes, for long periods of time, even that wasn't possible, and my housework was the only physical activity I had time for. My eating habits were erratic at best. I knew a lot about nutrition and working out; I just didn't have the time to implement it. If I felt some weight creeping on, it could usually be solved by some serious deprivation for a few days.

Then, as I approached and finally turned forty, I noticed a real decline in my metabolism and muscle mass. I was getting "skinny fat," meaning that I was slim but had no real muscle tone to speak of, and my metabolism was slowing to a crawl. While in the past, I had been able to get away with not always eating clean, now everything that I put in my mouth seemed to end up as fat somewhere on my body. Also, in the past, all I had to do was cut back on my calorie intake for a few days, and the pounds would come off; but even that was not working anymore! I realized that it was time for me to practice what I had learned.

At the same time, I had to face one of the biggest challenges of my life. My marriage of twenty-one years was over. This was a devastating and emotionally crippling time for me. After mourning the loss of my dreams and of my security and financial stability, I had to face reality and realize that I was now a single mom on my own. I could have let this "failure" define me and chosen to crumble. Instead, I slowly but surely gathered strength from knowing that I was living the life that I felt was the right one for me. I turned deeper and deeper into improving myself from the inside out. Working out became my "therapy." As I spent time in the gym and got physically stronger, I realized that I was also getting mentally stronger. With this newfound strength and the success I felt from advancing my health, I realized that I was indeed a capable person. My ex-husband had told me that I would never be able to succeed on my own or without him. But what I learned through the hard work on my physique and health was that I had all the tools I needed to indeed succeed and thrive on my own.

As I was in midlife, and knowing how important it is to maintain lean muscle mass, I implemented serious weight training combined with cardio and a real focus on my nutrition. As I started eating better and working out, I was learning what worked and what did not.

Eating boring and bland food is not necessary to lose fat and gain muscle.

Starving yourself definitely does not work. Deprivation does not work. Eating boring and bland food is not necessary to lose fat and gain muscle. In this book I will share with you what you should eat and how you should train so that while you will never be hungry, and you will not spend hours on end in the gym, you will be able to get into the best shape of your life, just as I have.

I now have a saying: "You can't out-train your diet." What this means is that no matter how much time you spend in the gym, you will not get the maximum results if you do not eat properly. Only working out and not paying attention to your eating is not going to cut it! Eighty percent of how we look and feel is determined by our diet. That's right, 80 percent!

So many people spend hours in the gym, only to undo all their hard work by not refueling their bodies correctly. Or even worse, they tell me that they work out so they can eat whatever they want. And then they wonder why they are still not feeling great or looking good.

In this book, I will share with you what you should eat and how you should train so that while you will never be hungry, and you will not spend hours on end in the gym, you will be able to get into the best shape of your life, just as I have done myself

One of my favorite sayings is that you have to "eat more to lose more." Sometimes, when people see me in person, they ask me, "Do you even eat? You must starve yourself to look like that!" But as I will share with you, nothing could be further from the truth. I will tell them that on most days while I was getting in shape, I ate egg whites and oatmeal for breakfast, and then I had a protein shake for snack a few hours later. Since I was still at work, I had another snack before I had my lunch of steamed tilapia, green peppers, and red onions. Midafternoon, I had a low-sugar protein bar, and for dinner I ate a delicious green salad with a homemade seafood gumbo. They look at me incredulously, because this is a lot of food. And I never allow myself to go hungry for long. I just don't like being hungry.

The secret lies in *what* we eat and *when* we eat. To lose weight, you need to use more calories than you eat, which is call a "negative energy balance." It is possible to eat any kind of food you want and lose weight as long as you are in what we call a caloric deficit. You need to limit the number of calories you eat every day and increase your daily physical activity. Portion control is imperative. Eating more often but smaller amounts of food, and choosing foods that are *naturally* low in calories but high in nutrients, are the keys to weight loss.

In this book, I will teach you how to enjoy five or even six meals a day, while boosting your metabolism to burn more fat and keep more of the lean mass that you have or will be building. You will drop pounds and get healthier for life. This is not a diet; this is a lifestyle change. You must be willing to commit to it for the long run, as any lasting change takes time. Soon you will come to prefer eating healthy foods and your body will thank you by getting thinner, leaner, and healthier.

Chapter 1: What Works?

Everywhere you look, there is advice on nutrition and what to eat. So how do we go about ensuring that we are eating right?

There are countless fad diets and even dangerous pills, injections, and other risky methods. None of these work in the long run. The fact is that severely-calorie-restricted diets often make you lose weight initially, but this is mostly water and (yikes!) muscle-mass loss. When you end up eating again, you will gain back what you lost, and MORE, due to the fact that you now have a slower metabolism and you lost muscle mass from all that dieting!

In the end, to lose weight and keep it off for good, you have to exercise at least five hours a week, and you have to eat more frequently but at the same time consume fewer calories than you burn to be at a negative energy balance, or *calorie deficit*, thereby loosing fat. That means that the food you eat must be *nutrient dense*, meaning high in nutrition per calorie. You do not want to waste your calories on food that doesn't make you healthier or protects you from disease—or worse yet, food that make you sick. *Everything* that we put in our bodies affects us in some way. It can be in a positive way or in a negative way. The choice is yours. You actually decide what you put into your mouth!

Even though there are many external factors that guide our choices, I want to make sure that you know how to make the best choice possible. This is why I have put together this plan for you. You will learn what it takes to make you the healthiest, leanest, and strongest you possible. The way I have come to the conclusions that I will share with you in this book is through a lot of schooling, much trial and error, and plenty of research. You no longer have to sift through all the confusing diets, workouts, and other information that is out there to try to figure out what is best for you. I have done this for you. Through my experiences with my clients and what I have tried myself, my family and I have been able to narrow down what really works and what does not. Now you are the one who will benefit, and I promise you that your body will thank you!

In this book, I will go over some of the basic themes of good nutrition that you can use to improve your body composition. I believe that it is important for you to understand the fundamentals of sound nutrition, so that you will know the *whys* of what I am telling you to do. One thing you will learn is that I don't really care too much about what you weigh, but what I do care about is that you have a healthy *body composition*. This is because what you should strive to do is to lose fat, not just weight! If you are at a "healthy" weight but your body fat is too high, I am not happy. This only means that you carry too little lean mass and too much fat.

You see, the scale only tells a small part of the story. You need to have enough lean mass to ensure that your metabolism runs efficiently. On the other hand, you may be overweight on the scale and at high risk for many diseases. You may be so desperate to lose weight that you try to starve yourself. Even though this is very difficult and unpleasant, it would most likely reflect an initial loss of weight on the scale. This can be encouraging, but it is not the weight I want you to lose. When you starve yourself, you lose muscle and water, not fat. This kind of weight loss is not only bad for your health, but it is also detrimental to your metabolism. You cannot sustain it, and in the end, you usually end up gaining back all the weight and more.

If you are tired of this kind of "yo-yo "syndrome, then you will love what I have in store for you. You see, my approach is not really a "diet" but a new way of life. I want you to lose *fat*, not lean mass or water weight. In order to do that, you have to *eat more to lose more* the safe and permanent way. And once you are at your goal weight, I will teach you how to stay there for the rest of your life.

Chapter 2: Your Metabolism

The one thing that determines the amount of food you can eat without affecting your weight is your *metabolism.* Your metabolism is the rate at which your body converts food into energy. The clinical definition of metabolism is "the set of chemical reactions that occur in living organisms to maintain life." It involves a complex network of hormones and enzymes that not only convert your food into energy but also affect how *efficiently* you burn that fuel.

Your metabolism is influenced by many different factors, such as your sex (men generally burn more calories at rest than women), your age (your metabolism slows about 5 percent per decade after the age of forty!) and your body composition, or how much lean mass you have. (The more muscle you have, the higher your metabolic rate tends to be.) Heredity and glandular function also play a role.

One way to *roughly* determine your metabolic rate is the following:

For a woman:

Multiply your current weight by 10. So if you weigh 130 pounds, your resting metabolic rate (RMR) would be roughly 1,300 calories.

The more active you are, the more calories you burn, so you must increase your calorie count accordingly. If, for instance, you get no exercise and only perform the basic activities of living, you are only moderately active. If that is the case you multiply by 10. If you exercise 3-4 times per week for about 45 minutes, you are considered moderately active. Then you would multiply your weight by 15. If you are a highly active individual and you do high intensity exercise on a daily basis for at least 45 minutes you may have to multiply your weight by as much as 18, so in this example the 130-pound woman would expend approximately 2,340 calories per day to *maintain her current weight.*

For a man:

Follow the same guidelines as a woman. But instead of multiplying by 10 you start with 11. A moderately active man would multiply his current weight by 11. So if you weigh 160 pounds, your RMR would be roughly 1,760 calories. Again, the more active you are, the more calories you burn, so you must increase your calorie count accordingly. If, for instance, you are a highly active individual, you may have to multiply your weight by as much as 18, so in this example the highly active man would expend approximately 2,880 calories per day to *maintain his current weight.*

The most accurate way to determine your actual metabolic rate is to obtain a professional measurement by a nutritionist or doctor.

As our metabolic rate is pretty mush set, what can you do to increase it? One of the most important things that you can do is to *eat more frequently.* Small but more frequent meals help put your metabolism into high gear and prevent the secretion of fat-storing hormones. In contrast, lowering both your calorie and fat intake decreases your metabolic rate. You need to eat at least five to six times per day to keep your body burning calories. Sounds like a lot, you say. Well, this is only three main meals—breakfast, lunch and dinner—and two to three high-quality snacks. Eating this way ensures that your metabolism stays elevated and you burn calories and fat throughout the entire day.

The worst thing you can do is to stop eating. We have all been there. You have a special event in a week, and you can't even button the top of your pants. Your first reaction is to stop eating. *What could be better?* you think. Well, actually, that is the worst thing to do simply because your body is designed through evolution to immediately start storing everything you do eat as fat in preparation for the next "famine." When you go too many hours between meals, your metabolism actually *slows down* to compensate for the lack of energy input. The longer you go without eating, the more of your "nonessential" body functions start shutting down. As you metabolism slows to a crawl, you feel and look sluggish and fatigued. You start craving "bad" carbs and sugar since your brain is low on glucose, and you are tempted not only to eat all the wrong things but also to overeat. Then, when you do eat, your new, slower metabolism burns fewer calories, and you may end up gaining weight more easily than you did before you went on a starvation diet. **This explains the so called "yo-yo dieting syndrome," where it becomes more and more difficult to lose or even *maintain* your weight.**

Instead, by eating small, frequent meals, you ensure that your blood-sugar levels stay stable and you never get too hungry. Your body will burn what you eat, and will also start to burn additional stored fat for fuel as you increase your activity level through exercise. There is no threat of "starvation," so your body continues to burn and your metabolism is actually elevated.

Think of it this way. If you have an open fire and you fail to put a new log on it, eventually it will burn out. If you add too big of a log (i.e., a huge meal), the fire can't burn either, but if you continuously put just the right amount of fuel, that fire will burn strong and bright. Your metabolism works the same way. In fact, research states that *any* food you eat will increase your metabolism, mostly within the first hour after you eat. This is due to the *"thermic effect of food,"* or TEF. This is the amount of energy expended by our bodies in order to process and digest food. Researchers at Georgia State University found that people who eat every two to three hours have less body fat and faster metabolism than those who only eat two or three meals per day. So, the more frequently you eat, the more you burn just by digesting and processing!

Chapter 3: Macronutrients

All foods are broken down into categories. There are macronutrients, micronutrients, and water. The three *macronutrients are protein, fat, and carbohydrates.* They all perform essential roles in our bodies, and they are the main components of our diet. They fuel our metabolism and it is therefore important to know which macronutrients you need and why. There are different qualities of macronutrients, and I will teach you which are your best choices in each category.We also require micronutrients such as vitamins and minerals, which will be discussed more in depth later on. All three macronutrients perform vital functions in our bodies and as such are needed in the daily diet.

Protein

Protein is the most important element of a healthy metabolism. Protein has four calories per gram, and about 35 percent of your calories should come from this macronutrient. The building blocks of protein are called amino acids. There are twenty different amino acids. Nine of these amino acids are considered essential, because our bodies cannot produce them naturally and therefore they must be supplied by our diet. Complete proteins are the ones that contain all twenty amino acids and are found in animal products such as meat, eggs, and dairy.

The crucial role of protein in the body is to maintain and repair muscle tissue. The more muscle you have, the higher your basal metabolic rate (BMR). So in essence, *protein is a great fat burner in that it speeds up your metabolism.* It is a critical component of a physically active person's diet, as it helps repair the damage to muscle tissue that occurs as you weight train.

Protein also has other roles. All enzymes are proteins and, as such, help your body digest foods. Proper digestion is critical for food absorption, weight management, and well-being. Hormones are also proteins. They tell your body through a system of signals, what to use for energy, and what to store as fat. When we eat the wrong kinds of foods, get stressed, or don't exercise or get enough sleep, our hormones can become unbalanced. When our hormones are out of whack, we feel lousy.

Finally, our immune system is aided by proteins, which help strengthen and repair cells. Protein also makes you feel fuller faster and longer since it slows down the rate of digestion. As you can see, protein is the main component of a healthy diet.

- **Aim to eat protein at every meal.**

Carbohydrates

Carbohydrates are the main energy source for the body. Like protein, carbohydrates also have four calories per gram. Your diet should consist of about 45 percent carbohydrates. Carbohydrates are chains of small, simple sugars that are broken down and enter the body in the form of glucose. Glucose is essential for the body in that it is the preferred source of energy for the brain, heart, and central nervous system.

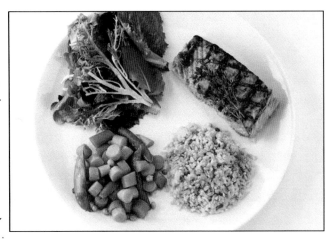

You should always choose complex carbohydrates, but what exactly are complex carbohydrates? The scientific explanation tells us that they are "complex compounds of three or more sugar molecules also called polysaccharides." Complex carbohydrates prevent too much sugar from being released into the bloodstream because they are high in fiber, which slows the breakdown and transit time. Fiber also helps prevent heart disease, the "silent killer" of women, and therefore plays an integral part of a disease preventing diet. Fiber also helps keep us "regular," which promotes greater intestinal health and in fact not only helps us feel fuller longer but also helps protect against many illnesses, including colorectal cancer. Fiber also helps regulate appetite, and most complex carbohydrates will keep you feeling fuller, longer, thereby reducing your cravings and hunger pangs.

Complex carbohydrates that you want to include in your diet are vegetables, fruits (in the morning), whole grains, and legumes.

In contrast, simple carbohydrates such as candy, sugar, soda and cookies are simple carbohydrates. These mono saccharides are composed of simple-to-digest, basic sugars with little real value for your body. The higher in sugar and lower in fiber, the worse the carbohydrate is for you. Simple carbohydrates, such as sugar, high-fructose corn syrup, and refined carbs, convert instantly to glucose, which is dangerous on two levels. First, your body can only carry a certain amount of glucose in the blood stream before the liver signals the pancreas to release insulin. When blood sugar levels rise too quickly, they are regulated to fall just as quickly, which leads you to the feeling of "crash and burn." Second, simple carbohydrates are more easily stored by the body as fat cells.

Do not eliminate carbohydrates. If you cut back on carbs too much, your body will be depleted of glycogen, the muscle fuel that gives you the energy to function. When you are not supplying the body enough carbohydrates to make glycogen, it has to make its own through a process called gluconeogenesis. Gluconeogenesis literally means "the making of new glucose". The body will make glucose from amino acids and glycerol (the backbone of triglycerides) At a certain point, something called ketosis will set in. For most people, consuming less than about 130 grams of carbohydrates per day will initiate ketosis. The body will produce ketones that trigger the conversion of fat to energy. This may sound desirable, but the problem is that ketosis is a dangerous state. While you are under consuming carbohydrates, the process of ketosis will convert fat to energy for the body to use. In severe cases, ketosis will cause headaches, mental fogginess, and bad breath along with many health problems including acid buildup in the bloodstream, which can be fatal.

In addition, cutting carbs too much also lowers the levels of serotonin in the brain. Serotonin levels are directly related to mood and anxiety. When your serotonin levels are too low, depression may set in. Another side effect of reducing carbs too drastically is that it affects your leptin levels. This causes your hunger to increase and your fat-burning potential to go down. Enjoy your complex carbohydrates in moderation to encourage fat loss while you maintain energy and focus.

- **Aim to consume the bulk of your carbohydrates early in the day, and then taper off. As you body's metabolic rate slows down naturally at night, preparing for sleep, you don't need carbohydrates.**

Fats

Contrary to what you might think, *fat is not always bad for you.* In fact, *fat is essential* for maintaining a healthy body and controlling your weight. The important thing is *what kind of fat* you are eating. Another thing to remember about fat is that it is *calorie dense.* With nine calories per gram, it is the most calorie dense of the macronutrients, and you must adjust your portion sizes to make sure that you are not getting too many calories from fat.

Your fat-loss diet should consist of about 25 to 30 percent healthy fat. Fats have many roles in the body, the main one being protection. Fat insulates to keep our body at the right temperature, and it provides cushioning to protect our organs. Healthy fats are necessary to your body for many other reasons as well: regulating hormonal production, improving immune function, lowering total cholesterol, lubricating joints, and providing the basis for healthy hair, nails, and skin. Fat enables the body to circulate, store, and absorb the fat-soluble vitamins A, D, E, and K. Without dietary fat, you would become deficient in these vitamins.

Finally, fat makes food taste better by adding texture, flavor, and aroma. Again, the key is to eat the right kind of fat. Remember, fat has nine calories per gram, almost twice as much as protein and carbohydrates, so as you can see it is important to watch the serving size.

Fats are broken down into two categories, *saturated and unsaturated.*

Saturated fats are found in animal products. Usually, saturated fats are associated with high cholesterol levels, atherosclerosis, and heart disease. Foods high in saturated fats that you should avoid are the following:

- butter, ghee, tallow, lard
- cottonseed oil
- palm oil
- palm kernel oil
- dairy products such as whole milk, cream cheese, and cream
- meat
- foods containing hydrogenated oils

Foods that come in packages are usually loaded with hydrogenated fat. Hydrogenated fats are also called *trans fats.* Trans fats are made in a process called hydrogenation, which uses hydrogen to harden vegetable oils. Trans fats raise LDL (bad) cholesterol in your blood and lower HDL (good) cholesterol levels. They should be *avoided at all costs* as they weaken your immune system, clog your arteries, break down your muscle, and foster chronic inflammation in the body, even causing some cancers.

Trans-fatty acids are found in commercially baked goods such as chips, crackers, donuts, and cookies and in many restaurant-prepared foods.

Healthy fats are the *unsaturated fats.* These are further broken down into polyunsaturated and monounsaturated.

Polyunsaturated fats have no negative effect on cholesterol levels. They include the following:

- safflower oil
- sunflower oil
- corn oil
- soy oil
- sesame oil

- fish oil
- omega- 3-rich fishes such as mackerel, salmon, albacore tuna, and sardines

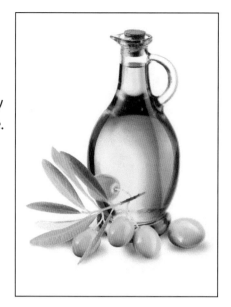

Monounsaturated fats have a positive effect on cholesterol by lowering LDL (bad) cholesterol, thereby preventing heart disease.

Monounsaturated fats include the following:

- olive oil
- peanut oil
- canola oil
- avocados
- all-natural nut butters and nuts
- flax seeds

Beware of "low-fat" or "fat-free" foods. They are often loaded with sugar and other artificial ingredients to enhance flavor, in effect making them highly caloric. Always check the label when choosing these products. These foods are not good options for better health and weight loss. It is significantly more beneficial to eat the natural fats we have discussed previously.

- **Fats can be consumed evenly throughout the day.**

- **Fats are calorie dense, so enjoy sparingly.**

Chapter 4: Micronutrients

Protein, fats, and carbohydrates are the macronutrients of food. The vitamins and minerals that are part of these foods are the micronutrients. They are essential to your health and make your body and central nervous system operate efficiently.

Vitamins

Vitamins are organic compounds. There are thirteen vitamins your body needs, of which four are called fat soluble.

Fat-soluble vitamins do not dissolve in water and are stored in your liver and your body's fat storage. They can build up and become toxic, so it is important to follow dosage recommendations carefully.

Fat-soluble vitamins are the following:

- vitamin A
- vitamin D
- vitamin E
- vitamin K

The water-soluble vitamins are the following:

- thiamin (B1)
- riboflavin (B2)
- niacin (B3)

Foods high in vitamin K include parsley, kale, spinach, Brussels sprouts, Swiss chard, green beans, asparagus, broccoli, kale, mustard greens, turnip greens, collard greens, thyme, romaine lettuce, sage, oregano, cabbage, celery and sea vegetables

- vitamin B-6, pyridoxine
- folate
- vitamin B-12, cobalamin
- pantothenic acid
- biotin
- vitamin C, ascorbic acid

> Broccoli, red peppers, Brussels sprouts, parsley, citrus fruit and strawberries are all high in Vitamin C.

Minerals

Together with vitamins, at least twenty-two minerals are needed by your body for optimal function and health. The most important minerals are listed below:

Mineral	What the mineral does	Effects of mineral deficiency	Good food sources
Calcium	Strengthens the bones and teeth. Also needed to help regulate the heartbeat and help muscle and nerve functions.	Its minor deficit can affect bone and teeth formation.	-milk -dairy products -green leafy vegetables -salmon -sardines -turnips -tofu -almonds -broccoli
Chromium	Required for the proper metabolism of sugar in the blood.	Can affect the potency of insulin in regulating sugar balance.	-beans -cheese -whole-grain food -peas -meat
Copper	Important for nerve functioning, red blood cell formation, and maintaining energy levels through iron absorption. Also good for healthy bones and the immune system.	Anemia, hair problems, dry skin, vitamin C deficiency.	-beans -raisins -chocolate -nuts -meat -shellfish
Fluorine	Helps to make bones and teeth stronger. Improves resistance to cavities.	Weak teeth and bones.	-gelatin desserts -saltwater fish (salmon) -tea -fluoridated water
Iodine	Helps keep your thyroid glands working. Your thyroid gland helps regulate the rate at which your body carries out its necessary physiological functions.	Enlargement of the thyroid gland.	-seafood -seaweed -dairy products -iodized salt

Iron	Helps the blood and muscles carry oxygen to the body.	Tiredness and lethargy, feelings of weakness, insomnia, palpitations.	-liver -red meat -egg yolk -legumes -whole / enriched grains -dark green vegetables
Magnesium	Helps muscles work, aids metabolism, and aids bone growth.	Fatigue, numbness, poor memory, muscle twitching and irritability, tingling, rapid heartbeat.	-whole grains -nuts -legumes -apricots -bananas -soybeans -green leafy vegetables -spinach
Manganese	Helps bone growth and cell production.	Rarely documented, one case showed in a patient a decrease in serum cholesterol, depressed growth of hair and nails, scaly dermatitis, weight loss, reddening of his black hair and beard, and impaired blood clotting.	-whole grains -fruits -vegetables -tea -egg yolk
Molybdenum	Helps cells and nerves to function.	Very rare, one observation has shown a patient to have developed rapid heart and respiratory rates, headache, and night blindness, and ultimately to have become comatose.	-dark green vegetables -peas -milk -beans -grains
Potassium	Essential for nerve function, muscle contraction, and maintenance of fluid and blood pressure in the body.	Depression, fatigue, hypertension, decreased heart rate.	-oranges -bananas -peanuts -beans -potatoes -spinach
Selenium	Helps to prevent damage to cells and aids in the functioning of the thyroid gland. An antioxidant for the body.	Poor heart function, osteoarthropathy, mental disability.	-brazil nuts -tuna -eggs -grains -chicken -shellfish -fish
Sodium	Helps to regulate water in the body's blood and tissue.	Fatigue, apathy, and nausea as well as cramps in the muscles of the extremities.	-table salt -dairy products
Zinc	Helps wounds to heal and aids taste and smell.	Growth retardation, hair loss, diarrhea, delayed sexual maturation and impotence, eye and skin lesions, and loss of appetite.	-whole wheat -peanuts -poultry -eggs -legumes -beef -shellfish

The RDA, or "recommended dietary allowances," sets standards from an expert committee. These recommendations list the average daily requirements for a variety of nutrients and are intended for healthy individuals.

Supplements

Supplements are nutrients that affect your body or metabolism in certain ways, and that you do not get through your regular diet or fluid intake.

There are countless supplements on the market today, and many claims on the benefits of all of them. It is confusing and can even be overwhelming to know what you need to take and why. Before you go out and spend a small fortune on supplements that you may not even need, I want you to read my suggestions. While none of these supplements are "magic pills" that will cause your body to lose fat all by itself, they do assist your metabolism to be the most efficient that it can be. I take certain supplements, and I will share the most important ones below. **Generally speaking,** all vitamins should be taken in the morning and minerals should be taken in the evening.

Vitamin C: Take at least one thousand milligrams. I personally take up to four grams per day of this powerhouse supplement, to protect my immune system, promote antioxidant activity in my cells, and even prevent chronic and inflammatory diseases such as heart disease and macular degeneration. Vitamin C is water soluble, so in case you take too much it is not stored in the body but will be secreted in your urine.

L-Carnitine: L-carnitine helps transport fat to the working muscle to use for energy. It stimulates the rate at which fatty acids are released into the bloodstream to be used for energy production. I take one gram per day to assist me in fat conversion to energy. Many L-carnitine products are now combined with raspberry ketones or green tea for even stronger fat-burning effects.

Glutamine: I take ten to twelve grams daily. Glutamine strengthens immune function and helps maintain muscle mass. It also helps recovery from exercise, promotes healing, and increases growth hormone levels. Glutamine is even used by doctors for its healing properties in cancer treatment. Glutamine should be taken one to two hours before training and *again* immediately after, for recovery. You can put it in your shake. I love glutamine!

Protein: To *increase* lean mass, I recommend as much as up to one gram protein per pounds of body weight per day. To *maintain* your muscle mass, you need to consume 0.6 to up to 0.8 grams per day per pound of weight. *In essence, the more active you are, the higher your protein requirements.*

Protein is necessary for the production of enzymes and hormones and vital in maintaining or building muscle. Eat it throughout the day at each meal. If you are going to supplement with protein powders, look for a low-carb, high-quality protein powder. Whey protein has been clinically proven to build muscle and enhance athletic performance. It has also been shown to help reduce body fat while at the same time increasing lean muscle mass. Wow! Another important benefit of whey protein is its ability to raise levels of IGF-1, a muscle-building chemical, while simultaneously decreasing levels of cortisol. Cortisol is an adrenal hormone that is secreted in response to stress. As you will soon learn, cortisol is also a fat-storing hormone.

Flaxseed: I recommend one tablespoon per day. Flaxseed is high in alpha linolenic acids (ALAs), an omega-3 fat, and fiber. These protect against cancers and cardiovascular disease, and increase digestive functions. Flaxseed is gaining more and more popularity due to its many benefits for health and body composition.

Omega-3: Take at least 1,100 milligrams per day. The benefits of taking omega-3 supplements *cannot be overstated*. Once in the body, they break down into *eicosanoids*. These are hormone-like substances that regulate the nervous system and immune response. Omega-3s protect brain function and work against coronary and other inflammation, regulate metabolism, help burn fat, regulate nervous system functions, and more. They can be taken at mealtimes.

Rhodiola Rosea: This is an adaptogen. Rhodiola increases energy and endurance, balances adrenals, and fights fatigue. Many women suffer from "adrenal exhaustion" due to chronic stress. I have found rhodiola incredibly helpful in treating this condition by balancing the output of the adrenal glands. Rhodiola also aids recovery and immunity. I give rhodiola to all my world-champion athletes, as it increases their athletic performance and endurance significantly.

Calcium, Magnesium, Zinc Complex: This trio helps support bone density while fighting off night cramps. Remember, calcium also decreases the amount of dietary fat that is absorbed by the intestines. It is believed that 70 to 80 percent of the population is deficient in magnesium, vitamin D, and zinc. Zinc is an immunity powerhouse. These supplements are all critical to and overall health. Take at bedtime for restful sleep; at least 1,500 milligrams of calcium and 750 milligrams of magnesium per day.

Vitamin D: Vitamin D protects against cancer, increases bone density by aiding in the absorption of calcium, and *is associated with greater muscle strength* by interacting with muscle receptors that activate genes for muscle growth and strength. Vitamin D is also associated with fat loss. Wow!

Probiotics: Our bodies are teeming with bacteria, both good and bad. Harmful bacteria can make us sick, while good bacteria help us stay well. Poor diet, stress, overuse of antibiotics, and other factors can create an imbalance in the body, where unhealthy bacteria overrun the healthy. Preliminary studies have not only connected the predominance of harmful bacteria to bad health but also to *weight gain*! Take probiotics daily.

Coconut Oil: I love coconut oil! Not only do I use it to cook with, I also put it in my shakes and pancakes, and I even eat it right off the spoon. Coconut oil has incredible benefits to your health and will be discussed more at length later in this book.

Chapter 5: How to Increase Your Metabolism

So, now you know what your metabolism is, what macronutrients and micronutrients are, and that you have to eat a certain amount of each of these five or six times per day to be healthy and promote fat loss.

Each individual has a given *resting metabolic rate*, RMR, due to factors such as age, gender, weight, height, and even genetics. This does not mean that you are stuck with the same metabolic rate forever. What are the things you can do to increase your metabolism?

There *are* ways to can change your basic energy requirements. As we discussed, your body can burn calories that come either from protein, fat, or carbohydrates. **The best thing you can do *is to boost your metabolism* so you can *eat more to lose more*. How can you do this?**

1. Eat Protein

Along with all the other benefits of eating protein that we already discussed, you need to know that *protein generally requires about twice as much energy to digest than carbohydrates or fats*. The amino acids in protein will lower the levels of stress hormone cortisol in the blood, which in turn boosts your metabolic rate. Eat protein with every meal!

Consuming whey protein has been shown to reduce the levels of ghrelin, which reduces hunger.

2. Exercise

Your body will burn fat through exercise. Fat on your body is essentially just that: energy that is stored for later use. So you have to use it to lose it! The great thing is that you will burn the most fat and require the most energy during the first two hours of intense exercise such as weight training or interval training. There is also an "afterburn" effect, which increases your metabolism for up to twenty-four hours after you work out. Maximize the calories you burn *and* the "after-burn" by adding high-intensity interval training (HIIT) into your workout. Alternate thirty seconds of all-out effort with ninety seconds of "recovery," or moderately paced activity. Do this ten times in one workout, and you will burn an additional one hundred to two hundred calories. Exercise is invaluable in weight loss and weight control.

3. Add Muscle

Every additional pound of muscle that you carry burns an additional fifty calories at rest per day, just to maintain itself. Never be afraid to gain muscle! Also, by adding muscle you prevent losing muscle weight. You will lose fat but maintain your muscle, which prevents a slowdown in your metabolism.

Remember that when you go on a starvation diet or stop exercising, your body responds by slowing down your metabolism and even by consuming its own lean mass for energy to survive. Women are often afraid to add muscle because they think they will get too "thick" or too "big." For a woman, this is very difficult if not impossible, due to a lack of certain hormones. You will not get bigger by weight training. In fact, studies show that you will get leaner and increase your RMR by adding muscle.

4. Balance Your Hormones Naturally

Hormones are chemicals that act as catalysts for changes in cells. They carry messages from glands to cells within tissues or organs in the body. They also maintain chemical levels in the body to help maintain homeostasis (a state of balance) in the body. When you control your hormonal balance, you will be that much close to controlling your weight!

There are two types of hormones known as steroids and peptides. I will go over the most important hormones that affect weight and hunger.

How Do Your Hormones Affect Your Weight?

The "Hunger Hormones"

Ghrelin: Grehlin is a twenty-eight amino acid peptide hormone that is secreted primarily by the stomach. Grehlin signals hunger to the brain and causes an increase in food intake. Unfortunately, grehlin levels have been found to increase when you eat fewer calories than your resting metabolic rate, and also when you eat too many calories. *When you skip meals or wait too long in between, levels of the appetite-stimulating hormone ghrelin start to rise.* Once those hunger pangs really kick in, you're likely to scarf down the first thing in sight. The key to keeping ghrelin levels low is to maintain as satisfied a feeling as possible.

Another trigger of increased grehlin levels is a lack of sleep. Studies show that people who sleep less than six hours a night experience an increase in grehlin secretion. *Being tired can make you fat!*

To keep grehlin levels stable, you should opt to consume the appropriate amount of calories throughout the day and get your ZZZs. Grehlin not only stimulates hunger; it also causes the increase of accumulation of lipids in the visceral fatty tissue located in the lower abdomen. This is the most dangerous type of fat tissue, associated with an increased risk for many diseases such as hypertension, high cholesterol, metabolic syndrome, and coronary artery disease.

Leptin: The other hormone associated with appetite is leptin. Leptin is produced by the fat cells in the body. *Leptin is known as an appetite suppressor* and has a direct impact on body weight and metabolism. Leptin helps signal the brain that the body has enough energy stores, such as fat. Unfortunately, obesity can make us resistant to leptin, so that even though we may have high levels of the hormone circulating in our bloodstream, we show impaired response. When leptin levels are too low, it signals the body to store fat. Again, sleep is directly correlated to the level of leptin in your bloodstream. Lack of sleep makes you hungrier as leptin levels fall. Also, it takes about twenty minutes for leptin to kick in after you start eating, so try to eat slowly, chewing (savoring!) your food completely before swallowing and stopping to drink water in between bites.

Peptide YY: This is a hormone that is released after eating. It acts with receptors to make you feel full and decrease your appetite. Wow! It also acts to slow down the movement of food in the digestive tract. Levels of peptide YY are highest two hours after eating. Conversely, when you starve yourself, or have certain illnesses such as celiac or Crohn's disease, you will suffer from low levels of peptide YY. These low levels are directly associated with an increase in appetite and food intake. It is therefore vital that you *eat more* to keep your levels of peptide YY elevated. Research also shows that *increasing your consumption of protein increases the release of peptide YY*, thereby helping reduce hunger and promote weight loss.

The "Fat-Storing" Hormones

Cortisol: The steroid hormone cortisol is produced in the adrenal cortex in response to hormones produced in the pituitary gland. Cortisol plays an important role in regulating blood sugar, energy production, the immune system, inflammation, and healing. Cortisol is released as a response to stress. The stress can be both physical and mental. Prolonged stress will result in chronically increased levels of cortisol in the blood stream, which leads to an increase in fat storage and weight gain. Yes, stress makes you fat!

To make matters worse, cortisol sends most of that stored fat directly to your middle, just to ensure your vital organs are safe. The key to keeping cortisol levels low is by adding some stress relief by doing something that you enjoy. *Remember, it is not selfish to take care of yourself!* You, as well as your loved ones, will benefit from your increase well-being, energy, and elevated mood. A healthy, happy you is a *better* you.

Insulin: Another peptide hormone that affects fat storage is insulin. We have already gone over many of the functions of insulin. Basically, insulin starts the process of converting sugar into cellular energy. It is produced in the pancreas and regulates glucose levels. Glucose comes from the food we eat, and insulin regulates glucose storage so it can be used as needed.

When you have more glucose (energy) than you need, insulin stimulates the liver and muscle cells to store it in the form of glycogen (energy for later use). Eating simple carbohydrates and other sugary foods stimulates the release of large quantities of insulin. As we know, the pancreas pumps it out to control glucose levels in the bloodstream and drive some of the glucose into cells. Blood-sugar levels drop again, resulting in hunger pangs. These fluctuations in insulin make you overeat and store fat.

If you often eat processed and high-sugar foods, your body can become less sensitive to insulin over time and you may develop something called *insulin resistance*. When you are insulin resistant, you require more and more insulin to convert the food you eat into energy for your muscle. Unfortunately, insulin resistance now affects 25 percent of the US population. It is the cause of fatigue, memory loss, mood swings, and more serious diseases such as type 2 diabetes, high blood pressure, stroke, and heart disease.

As you can see, keeping your insulin production at proper levels is critical for maintaining good health and body composition. So what can you do to maintain stable insulin levels? You have *to eat frequently to avoid swings in your blood sugar levels*, you have to eat whole grains and protein in favor of sugary, processed foods, and you have to exercise. Exercise also drive insulin levels down.

To keep insulin levels stable:

- Eat frequent, small meals.
- Avoid sugar and processed foods.
- Exercise.

Estrogen: Estrogen is a sex hormone that makes pregnancy possible and affects sexual function and metabolism. It is also affects mood and skin tone. Estrogen works together with progesterone, and both need to be in balance. *These two hormones help the body burn fat, control metabolism*, act as an antidepressant, and regulate sleep. Many women suffer imbalances as they enter perimeno-pause. Hormonal imbalances can also be caused by eating the wrong foods. Too much estrogen or estrogen dominance can cause weight gain, cellulite, and some cancers. Estrogen dominance can also cause anxiety, brain fog, low sex drive, and poor blood-sugar control.

You can avoid eating the foods that create estrogen dominance by eliminating processed foods and adding whole grains, fruits, and vegetables. *Fiber helps regulate estrogen build-up in the body*, so consuming high-fiber foods is very beneficial. The recommended daily intake of fiber is about fifty grams for an adult woman.

Progesterone: As you learned above, progesterone works in conjunction with estrogen. Progesterone burns calories and is a natural diuretic. It helps uterine fibroids, prevents cancer, improves mental clarity, and boosts libido. *Every month, progesterone levels plummet as you start ovulation.* Low progesterone levels cause cravings, insomnia, disrupted sleep, and daytime sleepiness.

Additional Supplements That Can Assist in Fat Burning

In addition to maintaining a balance on your hormones through diet and exercise, you can also add specific nutrients that have been shown to aid in fat burning.

Vitamin D: Thousands of studies on vitamin D have been completed over a span of forty years, and it's become clear that vitamin D is pretty incredible and effective. Rev up your metabolism and melt body fat by adding vitamin D and these five other natural fat melters.

Calcium: You already know that calcium helps you build strong bones and teeth. Calcium is also a wonderful mineral that works together with vitamin D *to help you shed fat.* Calcium is stored in fat cells. Research shows that the more calcium a fat cell has, the more fat that cell will release to be burned. Calcium also promotes weight loss by binding to fat in your intestines. This prevents some of it from getting absorbed into your bloodstream, where it can later be turned into stored fat.

Omega-3 Fatty Acids: As fat melters, omega-3s enable weight loss by triggering enzymes that increase fat-burning in cells. They also help boost mood, which may help reduce emotional eating. And omega-3s might improve leptin signaling in the brain, causing the brain to turn up fat burning and turn down appetite.

You almost can't consume vitamin D without consuming omega-3 fatty acids, and that's a good thing. Fatty fish like salmon (which is also high in D) are one of the richest sources of this beneficial fat. Other foods, such as nuts and seeds, contain a type of fat that can be converted into omega-3s after ingestion.

Monounsaturated Fatty Acids (MUFAs): MUFAs are a type of fat found in olive oil, nuts, seeds, avocados, peanut butter, and chocolate, and they have just one chemical bond (which is why they are called *mono*unsaturated). One Danish study of twenty-six men and women found that a diet that included 20 percent of its calories from MUFAs improved twenty-four-hour calorie burning by 0.1 percent and fat burning by 0.04 percent after six months.

Other research shows that MUFAs reduce visceral or belly fat. Specific foods that are high in MUFAs—especially peanuts, tree nuts, and olive oil—have been shown to keep blood sugar steady and reduce appetite, too.

Conjugated Linolenic Acid (CLA): CLAs are potent fat burners that are found, along with vitamin D and calcium, in dairy products. They are fatty acids that are created when bacteria ferments the food in the first part of the stomach of cows, sheep, and other ruminant animals. The CLA that is created through fermentation then makes its way into the meat and milk of these animals.

When we consume these foods, the CLA helps blood glucose enter body cells, so CLA can be burned for energy and not stored as fat. CLA also helps to promote fat burning, *especially in muscles, where the bulk of our calorie burning takes place.* CLAs can also be taken in capsule form.

Before you start super dosing yourself with all of these supplements and waiting for the fat to magically melt away, let me be clear: vitamin D and other fat melters *facilitate* weight loss, but they are not magic pills. If you just took a lot of supplements, you might see some effect. But to see real fat loss, you need to combine these supplements with eating the right way and exercising.

Chapter 6: How Do You Get to a "Calorie Deficit" to Lose Fat?

You have now learned what it takes to increase your basal metabolic rate, BMR, and what supplements you can take to facilitate fat burning, weight loss, and the increase in lean mass. The most important factor in weight loss is to be at a *negative energy balance.* Remember, this means burning more calories than what you consume. This forces your body to tap into its energy storage: your fat.

In order to lose weight, you need to know how many calories you should aim to consume per day. This is determined by your resting metabolic rate, or the amount of calories your body needs just to survive; the calories burned by exercise; and the thermic effect of food.

What Are Calories?

Calories are a measurement of heat. Specifically, one calorie is the amount of energy needed to raise the temperature of one gram of water one degree Celsius. The important word to take away from this definition is *energy*. Calories are energy that fuels our bodies, much like gasoline fuels our cars. Without sufficient calories, our heart would not beat, our lungs would not function, and our brain would not work. Many of us have no idea how many calories our body needs just to exist.

Remember, the rough way to estimate energy needs is to multiply your weight by the number ten. So if you weigh 130 pounds, you would need about 1,300 calories just to maintain your weight. Remember, though, that the more active you are, the higher the number you multiply your weight by will be. This is not an exact measure of your energy needs. A better, more accurate way to do this is to have it determined by a licensed professional such as myself, a doctor, or another type of health-care professional. In my practice I always determine my client's basic metabolic rate to be able to design a totally individual meal plan that will *ensure* that my client will lose fat.

If your goal is to lose fat, *I recommend a slow, steady, sustainable weight loss of about one to two pounds of fat per week.* Remember, one pound of fat is equivalent to 3,500 calories. So to lose one to two pounds of fat, you need to cut 250 to 500 calories per day and increase exercise by the same amount of calorie expenditure. Over a seven-day period, you can then lose one to two pounds of fat.

We are a society that wants instant gratification and results. Unfortunately, when you lose weight too quickly, you will most likely put it back on again. Research proves over and over that the safest and most *sustainable* weight loss is one to two pounds of fat per week. Be patient. It took some time to put the weight on. Now you must give yourself a chance to take it off and *keep it off.*

When you are cutting calories, you *must* do it the right way. By eating the right protein/carbs/fats ratio, you will feel full and satisfied. You will not crave sweets or want more food. You will also stimulate the production of the right kinds of hormones and enzymes to regulate your weight.

Now, eating the wrong ratio of protein/carbs/fats will leave you the opposite: feeling physically full but still hungry, not satisfied, craving sweets, and wanting to snack between meals. Your energy level and mood will also suffer when you are not eating the right way.

The macronutrient balance of our meals is vitally important. For fat loss, you should strive to get about 35 percent of your daily calories from complex carbohydrates, 45 percent from *lean* protein and 25 percent from healthy fats. Some of these requirements are also dependent on your present body type. Basically there are three body types: ectomorph, endomorph, and mesomorph.

- **Ectomorph:** This body type is lean with small joints and slight muscles. The physique is linear with long limbs. It is difficult for ectomorphs to build muscle, and they quickly lose fat.

- **Endomorph:** This body type is rounder or more "apple" shaped. The trunk is usually thick, and weight is carried in hips and abdomen. Endomorphs usually require a lot of cardio sessions to maintain their body weight. They do build muscle quite quickly though.

- **Mesomorph:** This body type is athletic and muscular. This body type builds muscle easily and appears symmetrical. Fat is evenly distributed on the body, and muscle mass is easily maintained.

Most people are a combination of two categories, such as meso-ecto or endo-meso. Each body type requires slightly different macronutrient ratios for fat loss. To best determine your exact body type and specific needs, it may be best to consult with a professional.

Now that we know the *ratios* of macronutrients that we have to eat, let's look at some samples of these macronutrients.

Protein

Our protein should be steamed, boiled, or baked. I never want you to eat your protein fried, breaded, or smothered in creamy sauces. *As I said before, protein is the single-most-important thing you can add to your diet.* It helps you retain or build muscle, and it reduces your appetite by keeping you full longer. Remember, you should aim to consume 0.8 to 1 gram of protein per pounds of body weight per day, especially if you are active. The USDA recommendation is only between 0.3 to 0.5 g per pound. Most fitness and weight-loss experts find this recommendation too low. The problem is that it's based on the needs of the *average* American. But every individual is different and therefore has different needs. In my practice, I have seen that people do much better when they consume more protein. Of course, too much of a good thing is simply that: too much. Excessive amounts of protein will not only cause weight gain; they may also put stress on the kidneys and liver.

Whenever you eat a carbohydrate, I want you to eat a protein. Protein serves to slow the digestive process, as it requires longer transit time in the intestines, thereby maintaining your blood-sugar levels and satiety. You should add lean protein to your diet by eating *fish, eggs, nuts, lean turkey, chicken, and soy products.*

Another great source of protein is *whey*. Whey protein has the highest levels of branched-chain amino acids of any protein source. BCAAs are an integral part of muscle development. Whey protein also stimulates fat burning and in study after study has been shown to assist in weight loss. Look for hydrolyzed whey protein, as this is the purest form of the protein, which contains the least amount of fat and carbohydrates and therefore is the most quickly absorbed.

- Aim for lean protein sources.
- Eat 0.8 to 1.0 gram of protein per pound of body weight.

Carbohydrates

We have already discussed the need for carbohydrates in the body. You must eat some carbohydrates to optimize your metabolic function. The difference is, which kind? Carbohydrates should always be "complex," meaning containing a lot of fiber, to ensure that your blood-sugar levels stay stable. An excellent example of a very low calorie, high fiber carbohydrate is vegetables. When choosing your vegetables, look for green veggies with high water content, such as lettuce, spinach, green beans, celery, and broccoli. For the highest nutrient composition, mix in colorful vegetables such as red and yellow peppers, tomatoes and shredded carrots, that contain high levels of antioxidants and minerals. In general, you want to

Studies show that people who eat fish at least twice a week have a 37 percent lower risk of heart disease.

look for carbohydrates that have low "glycemic index." The glycemic index measures how quickly ingested foods raise blood glucose or sugar levels. The higher the fiber content of a food, the lower the glycemic index usually is. Foods that have a high glycemic index value are more quickly digested and raise blood glucose levels faster. A high glycemic index diet contains foods such as sweets, white bread, pasta, potatoes, chips, and other simple carbohydrates. Eliminate these "white carbs," as they are refined, meaning most of the fiber has been take out of them, thereby causing a greater spike in your blood sugar levels when you eat them. Opt for the dark variety instead. Whole-grain breads, brown rice, and whole-wheat pasta are great choices.

If you love fruit, *the time to eat fruit is in the morning.* Fruit is certainly both nutritious and delicious, but fruit is also high in fructose, a natural sugar, which needs to be burned off through the day. *Fructose is a major trigger of insulin release* and will cause fat storage if not burned off. I cringe when I hear people say, "Oh, I eat really healthy. I only had a fruit platter for dinner." In terms of hormonal response, they might as well be eating donuts.

- Eliminate "white" carbs.
- Eat fruit only in the morning.
- Never eat carbs alone; always combine with a protein.

Fats

You must also add healthy fats to your diet. Remember that contrary to popular belief, fat does not make you fat; sugar does.

For years, other nutritionists and doctors preached the benefits of a low-fat diet. We were told that reducing the amount of fat we eat is the key to losing weight, managing cholesterol, and preventing health problems. Unfortunately, this has not proven to be true. "Fat free" is not a good choice for many reasons. *Fat-free or reduced-fat products are usually loaded with sugar and other chemicals to enhance flavor,* and that is not good for us. When it comes to your mental and physical health, simply greatly reducing or eliminating is actually harmful.

- We need to eat fat.
- "Fat free" is not better.

What Have We Learned So Far?

1. Protein and healthy fats control appetite and the rate of rise in blood sugar that helps control insulin. Therefore, eat protein at every meal and every snack, and eat some of the protein food first, before any carbohydrates, including alcohol.

2. The nutrient density of colorful vegetables and fruits is higher than that of most grain products, so get most of your carbohydrates from those colorful sources.

3. Most grain products made from flour of any kind tend to be *high glycemic index foods*. Consuming carbohydrates alone raises blood sugar quickly, unless you carefully follow rule number one and combine with a protein. Always chose complex carbs, which are those high in fiber.

4. Good fats are essential. Add a *few* unsalted natural nuts and seeds and a couple of teaspoons of high-quality oils or nut butters to your daily food selection. Watch the portion size of this calorie-dense food group.

5. Never, ever skip meals. Eat something approximately every three hours during the day. Do not let hunger be your guide as to when to eat. *Eat by the clock.* The two most common ways to slow metabolism are:
    - skipping meals
    - skipping exercise

6. Exercise at least five hours per week. Skip the long, boring cardio sessions and implement HIIT. The five hours should not all occur on the same day! Weight training is *the best* way to gain muscle, lose fat, and increase metabolism!

7. Don't expect to lose more than two pounds of fat per week. Anything more is not sustainable and will lower your metabolism in the long run.

8. Stay completely away from added sugar and sweetened foods. Eat as many natural food products as possible. If it comes in a box, be wary. Don't eat it!

9. Get enough sleep and cut down on stress. Remember, stress releases hormones that cause fat storage. Lack of sleep does the same!

- **If you overeat or neglect to work out, don't beat yourself up or use it as an excuse to stop altogether. Pick right back up where you left off and move forward.**

Chapter 7: Body Composition

I have told you that it is more important to monitor your *body composition* as opposed to monitoring your weight. *The scale only tells a small part of the story.* Many people, including some of my clients, mistakenly believe that just because the scale doesn't budge, they are not succeeding. I want you to remember that in the beginning of a new workout program, the body often retains water in the muscle cell as it is going through repair and healing. Just as your skin produces healing fluids to make a protective barrier when you cut yourself, the inside of your body does the same. So, sometimes you may not see an initial loss of weight on the scale. The important thing to remember is that you are improving your *body composition.* Eventually, you will see the number on the scale drop as your body adjusts to your new routine.

It is also important to remember that the same amount in weight of fat takes up much more space than the same amount of weight of muscle. *In fact, you may actually weigh the same, but take up much less space as you continue to replace fat with new lean mass.* As you can see in the picture, muscle is much more dense than fat, so it takes up less space even at the same weight.

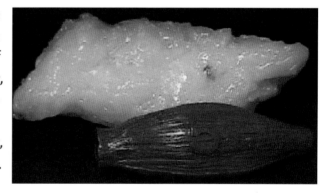

Your Perfect Body Fat Percentage

What is your perfect body fat ratio and why should you care?

Your body fat percentage is based on a few factors such as your weight, height, age, and gender. Below you will see a fat-percentage chart that divides BFP into several different categories.

ACE Body Fat % Chart		
Description	**Women**	**Men**
Essential fat	10-13%	2-5%
Athletes	14–20%	6-13%
Fitness	21–24%	14–17%
Average	25–31%	18–24%
Obese	32%+	25%+

As you see, the body-fat range varies greatly from men to women. It is important to note that women do need more body fat for reproductive function. We need to embrace our femininity and appreciate that we are not supposed to be as lean as men. Dropping too low in body fat will disrupt our monthly cycle and wreak havoc on our reproduction. As we age, women also undergo additional challenges in perimenopause and menopause, and retaining lean mass while fighting fat gain through impeccable nutrition and exercise becomes even more critical in stabilizing and maintaining a healthy body mass.

If you are female and have over 32 percent body fat, you are considered *obese.* A man is considered obese at just 25 percent body fat. Today, obesity has reached unparalleled proportions. Obesity is not just unsightly; it also carries tremendous health risks:

- Obesity is the second biggest cause of preventable death in the United States.
- Sixty million Americans twenty years and older are obese.
- Nine million children and teens ages six to nineteen are overweight.
- Being overweight or obese increases the risk of health conditions and diseases including breast cancer, coronary heart disease, type II diabetes, sleep apnea, gallbladder disease, osteoarthritis, colon cancer, hypertension, and stroke.

It is important to find a balance and strive to obtain a healthy body-fat percentage. You must feel what rate is best for YOU. Personally, I am pretty lean, and I like the way it makes me look and feel. Many people are surprised when they see me in real life, as I look more muscular in pictures. Wow, they say, you are much smaller in person. I am muscular but not *big*, as my body-fat percentage is low and I have well defined, toned muscle. To some, this look is too extreme, and they might want to aim for a slightly higher body-fat percentage. The one thing that is clear, though, is that we all want to avoid disease, so we must strive to maintain body fat levels in the healthy range.

There are so many benefits of being at a healthy weight and body-fat percentage. You will have greater energy, you will sleep better, you will look better and feel younger, and you will avoid developing major diseases and prevent inflammation, premature breakdown, and wear and tear on your body.

Chapter 8: Mental and Physical Preparation

So, now that you have decided to change your life and *eat more to lose more*, what are some things you should do before you get started on your new path to health? This chapter will give you a place to start.

Mental Preparation

Write Down Realistic Performance Goals

Never underestimate the power of the written word. Studies show that when you write something down, you are ten times more likely to actually carry through with it than if you don't write it. Buy a small notebook. On the first page you will write down your goal. Be specific. Instead of saying, "I will lose ten pounds" (which is an outcome goal), say "By this date, I will lose ten pounds *by* doing the following." Then spell out exactly what you plan to do. This is called a *performance goal*. One performance goal can be, exercising for forty-five minutes every Monday, Wednesday, Friday, and Saturday. Then do it!

Set *realistic* performance goals that you know are attainable. If you know that you only have twenty minutes to work out every day, then don't set yourself up for failure by promising yourself you will work out for an hour. Write it down, and then *stick to it.* By following your performance goals, you will achieve your outcome goal.

Studies show that people who set smaller, incremental goals for change succeed at a much higher rate than people who seek large, immediate change. We call them "baby steps."

Use Affirmations

Every morning when you wake up and every night before going to sleep, recommit yourself to your goals by saying this affirmation silently or aloud, *with feeling*:

I love myself, and I am worth taking care of. I will honor myself by eating clean, exercising, and staying positive. The more I give to myself, the better I, and those around me, will feel.

During the day, when you have a quiet moment, which may even be in the car, look into the mirror and *say out loud* to yourself: "I love you."

This may be difficult at first, and it may take some practice, but the more you do it, the easier it will become. It is essential that you develop this capacity for self-love. It is healthy and healing, and it will assist you in reaching your goal of being the best that you can be.

Visualize

Visualization is a very powerful tool. As a top trainer, I tell my competitive athletes to use the power of their mind to visualize performing flawlessly and to visualize themselves winning. Carefully construct and really "see" the picture in your mind of what it is you want to achieve. If you can "see" yourself in this way in your mind, you are actually creating the neural pathways for your body and brain to make it possible. *Practice visualization every day*. The more you see it, the easier it becomes to achieve it!

Avoid Limiting Beliefs

Most of our beliefs are operating on the subconscious level. We form our beliefs early on, from experiences and things we are taught about ourselves and others by parents and caregivers. Some of our beliefs are *limiting, and we may not even be aware of it*. They are part of our subconscious, but they still guide our everyday actions and choices.

You must examine how you feel about yourself and how you feel about food and exercise. If you recognize some of the common limiting beliefs, you can and must retrain your brain to accept beliefs that foster success.

Examples of limiting beliefs are:

- I hate being on any diet.
- I will try to eat better
- Exercise is boring.

- I will never be thin.

- I will always be heavy.

- I always quit working out.

- I will never be able to see my abs.

- My body works against me. I will never lose weight.

- I am too old to lose weight.

- It is too complicated to lose weight.

- I have no time to work out.

- I can't be so selfish.

- It's impossible for me to find time to work out.

As you will see, most limiting beliefs include extreme words like "try," "always," "never," "can't," and "impossible." If you recognize those words in your speech or thought pattern, it's time to take action and replace them with beliefs that foster success such as the following:

- I will...

- I can...

- I know...

- I am capable of...

- I want...

- I deserve...

- I believe...

Give yourself the power to succeed by eliminating limiting beliefs.

Be Realistic

Anyone who tells you it is easy to eat clean and healthy all the time is not really telling you the truth! Consistently eating right and sticking to your meal time takes a lot of *planning, discipline, and effort*. I have seen it in my clients, and I have seen it in myself! I have personally struggled, failed to plan, and also tried different methods that did not deliver what they promised. As I have tried to adhere to different eating plans, I have many times felt deprived, and although I may have lost some weight initially, it always seemed to come back on. I have been a vegan and a vegetarian, and I am now finally a "pescatarian," meaning that I eat fish but no other type of animal protein. I have tried low fat, low carb, the Zone Diet, the South Beach Diet, you name it. I have found, the hard way, through trial and error and lots of education, what works for me: eating limited portions of real food five to six times per day, prepared in my kitchen with real ingredients that are as unprocessed and unrefined as possible. This works every time. I never feel hungry or deprived, and I have been able to completely change my body composition.

I eat more than people think I do. When they see me, they often ask me how often I eat and what my meals consist of. I tell them I eat five times per day, and they cannot believe it. They have been led to believe that you have to starve or feel deprived to be lean, fit, and healthy. Quite the opposite is true. I eat every two and a half to three hours. *The key is* what *I am eating*.

I want you to know that it is *hard* to always eat right and stick to an exercise program. *You must be realistic.* Change takes time and tremendous effort. Our brains are hardwired to resist change and go back to what is familiar to us. You must repeat your new habits over and over until you become so comfortable with them that it no longer requires much effort. When you realize and accept this, you can overcome almost any obstacle. If you kid yourself into thinking that change is going to be easy, you will most certainly get frustrated and not succeed. *Recognize, accept, and embrace the challenge.*

Be Mindful

Mindfulness is being fully aware of the moment we are actually present in. We live in a world that is full of distractions and is a constant overload to our senses. Rarely do we get the luxury of doing one thing at a time and being present in the moment. We are expected to do many things at once, and this has unfortunate health consequences.

You should never feel guilty that you are doing only one thing at a time and actually paying attention to what you are doing. Think about how stress builds up during the day, as we try to do too many things at one time. *Many times when we eat our meals, we are not even aware that we are eating.* We may be driving our car while eating, or talking on the phone, watching television, working, or even grabbing food we see as we walk by. This is not only unhealthy but it also contributes to our feeling of not being full and satisfied. *We are not even noticing what we eat!* Being mindful will make you appreciate every bite that you put in your mouth, and savor the flavors of your food. While you focus on eating and really pay attention to every bite, you will feel full and satisfied like never before.

Try to make most meals a special moment to slow down and enjoy the process. Of course, we all have days when we have to eat on the run, and we grab whatever is available without much thought to either the food or the process of eating it. It happens to all of us. But it is important to try to get back to a slower pace of eating and a mindful way of enjoying our meals. I want you to try mindful eating, and you will see what it can do for you.

Stay Positive and Believe

Remember, sometimes you may lose your enthusiasm or optimism. This is normal. Changing old, ingrained habits takes a lot of work and focus. Research now shows that *it only takes five days (yes, only five days) to create the neural pathways for a new habit!* When you do something for five days straight, you have created a new habit! The problem is that your *subconscious* will always chose *old habits* over new ones, so you must stay committed until your "new habit" becomes your "old habit." By repeating your new habit and staying the course, you will succeed.

Recognize the difficulty and accept it. It is going to be hard sometimes, but it will be worth it. Remind yourself that you're really only taking a couple minutes' time out of each day in order *to remain committed and devoted* to your goals. Your future health and well-being is around the corner.

Here's what I've found from my experiences and from those of my hundreds of clients that I have counseled as well. If you start to stall, then take a step back and *recommit to your end goals.* Reconnect with that emotional feeling you had when you first started. Remember *why* you are on this journey. When you find that mental place, all of a sudden—and sometimes seemingly out of the blue—you *will* get a "second wind" of determination that will help you refocus. I promise you, there is a lot of inner work taking place, and old, emotions and habits may be resurfacing. Sometimes it may seem easier to quit. *Stay committed.* You can do this! You will do this! You will succeed!

Move Forward

There may be times when you are not able to follow the meal plan or workout program. Due to stress, illness, emotional issues, boredom, travel, or maybe just plain hunger, you may have bad days where you can't seem to control your eating. The key in this situation is to *stay the path.* Do not use one bad meal or bad day as an excuse to stop the progress and slide back into old habits. Recognize that *no one is perfect all the time* and that you are only required to *be persistent, not perfect.* Pick right back up, and don't berate yourself. That only creates more stress and anxiety. Remember that today is the first day of the rest of your life, and every moment is a chance for a new beginning. Get back on the program and *smile.*

Develop a Support System

Sometimes when you are trying to change your old habits for new or better ones, your friends and even your family might undermine your efforts. This can be due to fear, jealousy, or just plain ignorance. At those times, it is important to remember your "end goal" of better health so you won't give in to their pressure. When faced with a friend who keeps nagging you to eat something that you don't want, tell him or her you'll try it later. This usually satisfies people for the moment, and then they will forget.

Also, you may just have to learn to stand your ground and develop your "mental muscle." As women, we are taught to be "nice," and often we think that means saying yes to everything that comes our way. Practice saying no, and don't feel bad about it. If you stick to your guns, you will build support and gain respect, and you may even motivate your friends and loved ones to join you in your quest for better health. You are doing everything you can to make yourself a better person, inside and out.

If you have a bad day, or week, don't berate yourself and give up. *Giving up is not an option.* Always recognize what happened and why you gave in so you can learn from the experience. It could be stress at work, PMS, emotional eating, a birthday celebration, you name it. I have heard it all! *Get over it and get back on track.* No one is perfect all the time. Recognize your challenges and plan accordingly. "Persistence, not perfection" is one of my favorite JNL quotes. And it's true! Don't make excuses: make plans and stick to them.

Physical Preparation

Even though you probably can't wait to get started on your "eat more to lose more" plan, there are a few things you should do first to ensure your success.

Take "Before" Pictures

It is important to take pictures to record your progress. You will see yourself in the mirror every day and may not recognize the changes that are taking place in your body. Having pictures to compare is a surefire way to see the real transformation that will happen.

Here is how to take your "before" picture:

Front View: Stand up straight with your feed hip-width apart. Arms are at your sides but off your hips, so you can see the shape and width of your hips.

Front View with Pose: Same as above but flex your biceps in a classic weight-trainer's pose.

Side View: Stand up straight, arms hanging down at your side. Make sure your hands are in the middle of your thigh. You don't want your hand blocking the outline of your thighs or glutes.

Back View: This pose is much the same as the front view, but with your back to the camera.

Back View with Pose: Same as front view with pose. You want to show your upper-back definition here.

Upload the photos to your computer and place them in a folder marked with the date. Also, create a document listing the date, your weight, and your measurements.

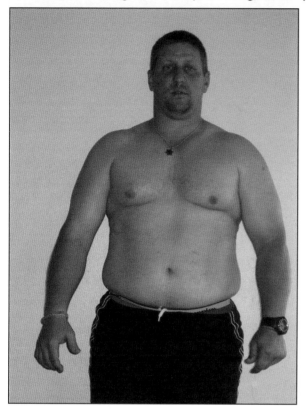
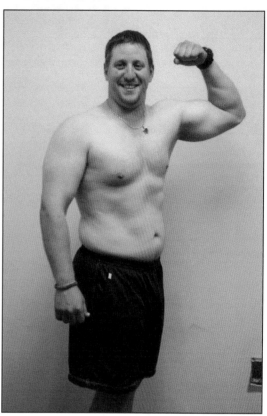

Before   After

Julio lost twenty-six pounds of fat in eight weeks while following the Eat More to Lose More Program.

Rid the Pantry

Throw out or give away all foods that are not on the meal plan and that will stand in the way of your success. If you think that you need to keep processed, sugar-laden, artificial foods in your home for any reason, *you are wrong*. No one in your family, including your kids, benefits in any way from eating or drinking that stuff. Why keep it around to tempt you into eating it? *Don't give temptation a chance.* You will only get grumpy and feel deprived looking at things that you should not eat. Get rid of it!

Go Grocery Shopping for Must-Have Staples

Lean Protein

- lean fish, such as tilapia, halibut, cod and snapper

- chicken and turkey to be grilled, baked, or boiled—never fried or breaded.

- albacore tuna, to be rinsed with water and drained before serving, then seasoned with lime, lemon, and spices, *not* mayo (Due to high mercury content, tuna should only be enjoyed twice per week.)

- salmon, to be eaten once or twice a week by oven baking, boiling, or steaming (Try buying the wild-caught kind.)

According to the USDA, adding lean fish to your diet can increase your intake of healthy fats. One 3-oz. serving of cod provides only 89 calories, with 19 g of protein.

- eggs, mostly whites, one or maximum two yolks per day (Try liquid Egg Beaters or All Whites.)

- low-fat Greek yogurt, unsweetened (Fage plain is a good choice.)

- low-fat cottage cheese, organic. (The small, snack-sized cups are great for portion control.)

- protein powder supplements (Try to find the ones made by reputable companies. Make sure that your protein powder contains no more than four to five grams of sugar per serving. I recommend Max Muscle, Dymatize, or BSN products.)

Vegetarian Protein Sources

As you know, I am a fish eater, but I do not eat any type of meat. Many people ask me how I am able to meet my daily protein requirements by eating this way. I tell them that I get plenty of protein from fish, seafood, protein supplements, and also vegetarian protein sources. I tend not to eat vegetable protein products frequently, as it does contain a lot of carbohydrates per gram of serving, and as such I classify it as carbohydrates, not protein.

1 cup red bell peppers contain 152 mg vitamin C, 3,726 IU vitamin A, and 251 mg potassium.

You will find vegetarian and vegan dishes in my recipe section that include some of the following;

- seitan

- soy

- tofu
- tempeh
- texturized vegetable protein

Today, it is easy to find almost any vegetarian substitute for real meat. Eating less red meat is essential in your quest for better health.

Veggies

- spinach
- mixed lettuces, arugula, kalecucumbers, celery, radishes
- tomatoes, bell peppers, carrots
- cruciferous veggies such as broccoli and cauliflower
- green beans, asparagus, kale, Brussels sprouts
- Veggies can be consumed at every meal! I eat a large amount of organically grown greens each day.

Fruits

To be consumed in the a.m. only

- mixed berries, strawberries,
- raspberries and blueberries (These are a great choice, as they are loaded with antioxidants.)
- cherries
- bananas
- apples, grapefruit, and oranges

Cherries are loaded with antioxidants and anti- inflammatory properties!

Complex Carbohydrates

- sweet potatoes or yams, to be eaten baked or boiled, *not* mashed with butter or fat
- brown rice
- whole-grain pastas
- quinoa (This is very high in protein.)
- oatmeal, unsweetened
- beans and legumes in limitation

- low-sugar cereals or granola
- low-sugar, whole-grain waffles
- low-sugar, whole-grain breads (I recommend Ezekiel Bread, which contains no artificial ingredients or preservatives.)
- low-carb, whole-grain tortillas
- low-carb pita pockets (These are great to stuff with a lean protein ahead of time as a take-a-long snack or meal.)

Fats

- roasted, natural, unsalted nuts or nut butters
- avocado (1/8 avocado = 1 serving)
- olive oil
- coconut oil
- fish oils
- flaxseed
- cooking spray made *without silicone* (Please read the label!)
- reduced-fat mayo
- pesto sauce
- hummus

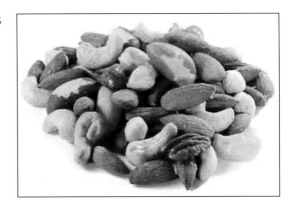

Drinks

- water
- green tea (a natural fat burner)
- herbal tea
- unsweetened iced tea
- coffee in the morning or before a workout

People who drink three cups of coffee per day have a 10 percent chance of living longer than non-coffee drinkers.

Seasonings

- salt-free Ms. Dash in all different varieties
- hot sauces
- lemon, lime
- salsa
- onions, garlic
- fresh herbs

Sweeteners

- Stevia

Stevia is an all-natural, zero-calorie sugar substitute from a South American plant. Stevia is safe for diabetics and assists in regulating blood sugar. It is now being used in some diet sodas, instead of *artificial sweeteners that actually may cause cancer in addition to making you crave more carbohydrates.*

Invest in a Food Scale

Most people *grossly miscalculate* the correct size of a serving. Until you learn what, for example, four ounces or half a cup looks like, *use a food scale or measuring cup*! The more you use it, the quicker you will learn what these units of measurement actually look like in real food. Then you will be able to more correctly eyeball serving sizes.

Generally speaking, these are guidelines to eyeballing serving sizes:

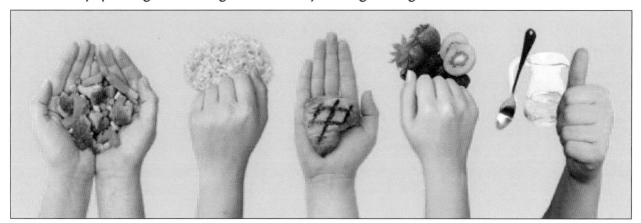

- Protein should be the size and thickness of your palm (no fingers).
- Carbohydrates should be the size and thickness of your hand including fingers.
- Fats should be the size of your thumb.

Keep a Food Journal

Many studies show the power of recording. People who write down or journal what they eat and drink actually lose more weight than people who don't keep a food journal, and they keep the weight off! Write down or use an app on your smart phone to record everything you put in your mouth.

Additionally, if you are an *emotional eater,* recording your present mood as well as what you eat and drink may help you detect and overcome certain patterns that are standing in your way of success. Go back to the section on limiting beliefs and recheck your thought patterns. Believe!

Chapter 9: Exercise

I t is imperative that you exercise at least four to five times per week. The US government now recommends that we get five hours of exercise per week! You must divide these hours up. Don't expect to gain the same results from working out for two to three hours on the weekend and doing nothing all week. It is so much better to do thirty to forty-five minutes almost every day. And, if twenty minutes is all you have, then do that. It is always better to do something, even if it's less than you want, than to do nothing at all.

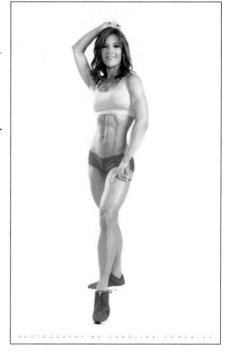

PHOTOGRAPHY BY CAROLINA GONZALEZ

Try Interval and Weight Training Combined

Studies show that people who engage in interval training boost their metabolic rate not only *during* exercise but for up to fourteen hours after they stop working out! You will burn twice as many calories by interval training than by steady pace training. Try doing a one-minute full-effort activity followed by a two-minute recovery period, such as running then jogging, and repeating for eight to ten times.

When you add strength training to your routine, your metabolic rate will also be elevated. Try the JNL Fusion method. This revolutionary system combines *both* interval training and strength training for unparalleled results! I train myself with this method, and I also train my clients this way. Combining weight training with thirty-second cardio "bursts" between sets gives me the fat burning *and* the muscle building that I want to achieve in one quick, super-efficient workout.

47

As we age and our metabolism naturally declines, it becomes even more important to incorporate strength training in our routines. Your metabolism declines 20 percent between the age of forty and sixty. As you incorporate weight training, you will see increase not only in lean muscle mass retention but also in prevention of osteoporosis or bone-density loss. Do not fear weight lifting, as it is the best thing you can do to maintain a youthful, healthy body and stoke your metabolism at the same time.

My clients ask me again and again: What's better, weight training or cardio? Hands down, weight training wins. But if you add the cardio in between sets as well, you have a surefire winner.

Weigh Yourself Once a Week

Keep track of your progress by weighing yourself. I want you to weigh yourself *only once a week*. Do not step on the scale more often than that! Your weight fluctuates throughout the day, depending on the food you eat, your hydration status, what time of the month it is, and other factors. If you weigh yourself every day, you may find that you fluctuate a lot, and that may set you up for an emotional roller coaster.

Instead, weigh yourself once a week, always at the same time, wearing similar clothing each time. I weigh my clients each week and check their body fat, to measure progress. You can invest in a scale that gives you a body-fat readout, but they are not always reliable. The most accurate body-fat measurements are obtained by a professional such as a trainer or nutrition specialist. You can also buy a caliper and record your own measurements.

Sometimes when you start an exercise program, you may not see a drop in your weight. It is therefore important to measure your body fat, as you may indeed be losing fat and gaining muscle, showing an overall weight gain or lacking the loss you may be looking for even though you are improving your body composition.

Avoid Overtraining

Just as it is important not to starve yourself, you must also avoid training too much or too hard. Sometimes, when we start a new lifestyle or want to reach results quickly, we tend to go to extremes. We get so excited that we jump in with both feet, and we want to see quick results so we train more than what is called for.

Unfortunately, with training, more is not always better. Your body needs to recover from exercise and have time to repair. Working out is, in fact, a stressor on your body, as you are actively breaking down or tearing muscle fiber and putting stress on your cardiovascular system. This is why it's so important to allow for at least one day of complete rest. If you ignore your body's need for rest, you will actually start to break it down, causing fatigue, disturbance in appetite, or even worse, frequent colds and other illnesses. So, as much as you want to achieve your goals as quickly as possible, remember to respect your body's need for rest and repair. Lasting change takes time. Be patient.

The Sunday Ritual

Fail to prepare and you prepare to fail! It's been said before, and it is true. Preparation is really the key to success. The way I have incorporated this into my life is by doing something I call the "Sunday Ritual." Quite simply, Sundays are the least busy days for me, so I have the time to go to the grocery store to buy my fresh and natural staples, and then I have the time to prepare them in bulk when I get back home.

I cook large quantities of brown rice and bake sweet potatoes in the oven that I can reheat later. I clean and marinate fresh fish in lemon juice and spices and store it in the fridge for a meal that's ready in minutes. I clean and chop vegetables for my salads or for use in omelets. I marinate and grill

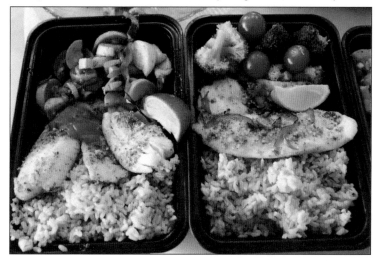

chicken in bulk so that it's ready to go to work or school or be eaten for dinner at a moment's notice. I make and store turkey burgers so they're ready in a snap. I drain and rinse canned albacore tuna, then season it with lime juice and fresh salsa for a delicious salad topping or pita pocket stuffing.

The few hours that I spend in this ritual are well worth it. This ritual prevents me from grabbing the wrong kind of food when I am starving and pressed for time. It allows me to send healthy foods to school with my kids or to pack a great lunch for Willie or myself in no time. It even gives me a little more time to relax in the evening after a long day at work, because my staples are already cooked and I can quickly put together something delicious and satisfying.

Find a day when your schedule permits this kind of preparation. You will love it! You can even ask other family members to help you, as this is great time spent together.

Willie and I make food trays on Sundays to have healthy lunches ready to go during the week.

Let's look at my most important Tips for Success

- Eat every 2.5 to 3 hours, hungry or not! Set an alarm on your watch or smartphone to remind you when to eat to eat.

- Try to eat your meals at the same time each day.

- Do not eat carbs alone; always combine with a protein.

- Drink at least seventy fluid ounces of water per day.

- Shop the perimeter of the supermarket; the middle is filled with processed, artificial items.

- Prepare staples such as grilled chicken, turkey, and fish on Sundays and store in the fridge.

- Stock your fridge and pantry with healthy snacks, and throw out foods that are bad for you.

- Do not use added sugar.

- Use added salt sparingly.

- Season with sodium-free products and natural spices, citrus, and salsa.

- Carry snacks with you if you know you are going to be out for more than two hours.

- When dining out, don't hesitate to be specific while ordering. You are the paying customer!

- Carry your supplements and protein powders with you to drink within thirty minutes post workout.

- Exercise at least forty-five minutes per day, five to six days per week.

- Skip alcohol.

- Avoid artificial sweeteners that only add to your cravings.

- Keep a journal where you track your food and exercise.

- Write down your goals.

- Rest at least one day per week.

Chapter 10: Food Specifics

A Word about Sugar

One of the biggest hurdles people face in their diet is consuming way too much added sugar. When we consume added sugar, we are not getting the nutrients that we need. Sugar adds unnecessary calories without adding beneficial nutrients. You may not even know how much sugar you are eating! Did you know that the average American consumes about 150 pounds of added sugar per year? If you regularly drink soda, by just cutting *one* can per day you will lose fifteen pounds in one year.

On average, Americans consume 150 lbs. of added sugar per year!

Cutting just one soda a day can result in a weight loss of 15 lbs. in a year.

Even foods that we do not consider "sweetened" actually contain a lot of added sugar. These include bread, yogurt, crackers, cereals, juice mixes, and much more. *Read your labels*. You want to stay away from things that have calories from sugar greater than 20 percent of total calories. That means that a one-hundred-calorie item should have a maximum of five grams of sugar, as each gram of sugar has approximately four calories.

Sugar also stimulates the release of *insulin* from the pancreas to regulate blood sugar levels. We already talked about how this hormone makes you store fat. When blood sugar levels drop, *cortisol* is released from the adrenal glands. Remember that cortisol is a fat-storing hormone that is also released during periods of stress. *Sugar stresses the adrenal glands.* As you can see, it's a vicious cycle. So, there is really no benefit to sugar. It does make your food taste sweeter, but if you stay off sugar for just a few days, you will develop new, healthier taste preferences.

Sometimes, in our avoidance of real sugar, we may think that artificially sweetened foods are better for us. *Unfortunately sugar-free or sweetened with alternative sweeteners is not necessarily better.*

A lot of *artificial sweeteners* have come under scrutiny for ailments ranging from migraines to cancer. Also, when we give our bodies sweetened foods, it actually tricks our brain into craving *more* sweets.

I suggest cutting down or eliminating sweetened foods completely. It takes the body about five days to get rid of a sugar addiction. You may be miserable for the first few days, getting headaches and feeling very deprived, as the body goes through withdrawal much as it does with a drug addiction. Yes, a real drug addiction. That is because sugar is just as addicting as some other drugs, and you will go through withdrawal!

If you can do it, and you get through this stage, you will actually feel better; and if you try sweetened foods, you will notice that you find them much too sweet. More importantly you will actually not crave them so much anymore.

Sometimes sugar is not listed as sugar on a label. There are other ways for food manufacturers to add sweetness that you need to look out for. **If the label has one of the following ingredients, skip it!**

- brown sugar
- corn syrup
- dextrose
- fructose
- fruit juice concentrate
- glucose
- honey
- lactose
- maltose
- molasses
- raw sugar
- sucrose

A Word about Diet Sodas

Drinking diet soda or other artificially sweetened drinks to avoid calories *may* sound like a good idea, but in reality it tends to come along with other behaviors that may endanger your health. "Although our data did not clearly support this theory, I suspect that persons drinking diet soda are likely eating other foods that elevate risk of metabolic disorders," says Jennifer Nettleton, PhD, assistant professor of epidemiology at the University Of Texas School Of Public Health, in Houston.

"People drinking diet soda are likely to miscalculate the amount of caloric savings, thus over-consuming other foods, resulting in greater overall energy consumption." There is also research showing a link between consuming artificially sweetened foods leading to an *increase* in cravings for more sweets. Additionally, diet soda is 100 percent artificial and contains absolutely nothing that is good for your body or your health. Nothing!

Here's how to avoid the health problems that come in a soda can:

Drink water. Hands down, *the best thing you can drink is water.* Being well hydrated not only makes you feel better as well as perform better in the gym, it also elevates your metabolism and increases other functions such as joint lubrication and digestive functions. It even gives you shiny hair and glowing skin. A new study in the *American Journal of Clinical Nutrition* found that switching from sugary drinks to water can lead to a weight loss of 5 percent of your body weight or more in only six months!

Want to add some flavor to your water? Add slices of lemon or lime, mint leaves, or slices of apple and strawberries.

Drink green tea. Another metabolic booster, *green tea increases fat burning*, prevents obesity, and lowers levels of blood sugars and fat. Hydrate with green tea, and reap the antioxidant benefits of this great health booster.

Green tea's many health benefits stem from the high contents of antioxidant flavonoids. These halt oxidative damage to our cells and protect us from cancers and heart disease.

A Word about Red Meat

Limit or severely cut back on eating red meat. A new study from Harvard University finds that the more servings of red meat you eat per day, the higher your chance of dying over a twenty-year span. This risk increases by 12 percent with each additional daily serving. Meat has high amounts of saturated fats and, sadly, today contains *hormones, antibiotics, and other substances that are harmful to our health*.

If you must indulge in red meat once in a while, please consider buying the grass-fed kind, as it is much less loaded with toxins and other remnants of conventional farming. I have not eaten red meat ever, so it's a myth that you need it to stay healthy or to build quality muscle. I have also never experienced anemia, not even in my four pregnancies, so it is also a myth that you must eat red meat to get sufficient amounts of iron.

A Word about Dairy Products

I eat very little dairy, and here is why: unfortunately, today, dangerously high levels of artificial hormones, antibiotics, and other toxins are found in commercially produced dairy products.

One of the worst substances, dioxin, is highly toxic, according to the World Health Organization. Dioxins cause reproductive and developmental problems, damage the immune system, disrupt hormones, and cause cancer. Dioxin will build up in your tissue and can stay there for years before you feel any ill effects. My advice is to avoid products that are known to contain dioxin.

When purchasing dairy products, ALWAYS opt for the organic kind as conventional dairy products are loaded with harmful chemicals and residues.

I have also found that when I eat a lot of dairy, I get bloated and build up a lot of mucus. If you are concerned about getting enough calcium and vitamin D without eating dairy products, you need not be. You can get both from leafy greens and the natural foods that will be included in your meal plan.

A Word about Alcohol

Alcohol has no place in a weight-loss diet. The effects of alcohol can be detrimental to your weight-loss success as well as to your overall health. Alcohol diminishes performance, affects mental clarity, and can create addiction and even diabetes and liver disease.

When you drink alcohol, you are consuming "empty" calories, or calories without nutrition. You are also reducing your body's ability to burn fat. The liver, which has to process the alcohol immediately, as it recognizes it as a toxin, cannot simultaneously stimulate other fat-burning mechanisms. When you drink alcohol, your fat burning can go down by as much as 30 percent. While you are drinking alcohol, this is the first energy that the body will burn. Any other fat burning simply will not take place. So the effect on your diet is not just the calories that you consume from the alcohol but also the *reduced fat burning* caused by alcohol consumption.

Alcohol also lowers you inhibitions. This can spell disaster as your willpower vanishes and you find yourself throwing your meal plan to the side and reaching for all the wrong foods. *At seven calories per gram, alcohol supplies almost twice as many calories as protein and carbohydrates.* You do not need alcohol, and drinking it will not benefit your body positively. Although there are health benefits from drinking one glass of red wine per day, I have found that while on a weight-loss plan, my clients do not do well when they include this daily glass of wine. It would be better to enjoy this glass of wine when you have reached your goal and stayed there for a good month or more.

A Word about Coconut Oil

I love coconut oil and use it daily. Coconut oil is high in lauric acid, a medium-chain triglyceride (MCT) that helps boost immunity, shed belly fat, and ward off digestive issues. Medium-chain triglycerides are absorbed directly from the intestines into the portal system and sent to the liver instead of the lymphatic system, as other fats are. This prevents them from being stored as fat and instead makes them available to be used for immediate energy needs.

The health benefits of coconut oil are almost endless. They include hair care, skin care, cholesterol management, weight management, better digestion, and relief from heart disease, high blood pressure, diabetes, and cancer. There is also evidence that a diet rich in coconut oil can improve the symptoms of HIV, ADD, and autism.

Also, coconut oil has been shown to have anticancer, antiviral, and antifungal properties as well as doing wonders for your hair, nails, and skin. The important thing to remember, though, is that even though coconut oil is a veritable health food, it is still a fat and, as such, high in calories. *The best use for coconut oil is in a low-carbohydrate diet,* where the body will not convert the coconut oil to stored fat but to energy for immediate use.

A Word about Eating Out

I know from my own experience as well as that of my clients that eating out can be very difficult while trying to lose weight. It can seem almost impossible to resist the delicious, fat-storing foods that are on the menu and all around you. You will definitely have to use your mental power to stay focused on your health and not fall into temptation.

I can tell you, though, that it is entirely possible to stay on the meal plan, while eating out. You do not have to cut your social life or family or work events just because you are on this weight-loss program. Indeed, in today's health-conscious society, most restaurants are more than willing to serve you a special order of steamed or grilled chicken or fish with a side order of vegetables. The secret is to be *very specific* when you order. If you tell servers in a nice way that you have special dietary restrictions, they are usually more than happy to accommodate you.

In addition to ordering what you would normally eat at home, there are a few more tips that will help you stay clear of unwanted calories and fat.

- Drink water as your beverage.
- Skip the bread basket.

- If you order salad, get the dressing on the side and make sure it is vinaigrette.
- If you order soup, skip the creamy one and get a vegetable-based soup.
- Skip dessert.
- Don't go to the restaurant starving. Plan ahead and eat normally up to three hours before your restaurant meal.

A Word about Chromium

Chromium is a trace mineral that is not often associated with the human body. However, because it directly affects many components of weight management, many dieters have been exploring the role of chromium, specifically its form as the supplement *chromium picolinate.*

Chromium is indeed useful as it does the following:

1. aids in the regulation of blood sugar metabolism

2. promotes storage of energy reserves in the body

3. regulates hunger and reduces cravings for food

4. controls blood levels of cholesterol and fat

5. promotes proper functioning of the central nervous system

The recommended daily intake of chromium is twenty to thirty-five micrograms per day, but the maximum is three hundred micrograms daily for those who take chromium picolinate as a weight-loss supplement.

Foods that are particularly rich in chromium are *brown rice, whole wheat and other whole grains, whole-grain products such as whole-wheat bread and rye bread, Brewer's yeast, eggs, cheese, turkey, fish, oysters, mushrooms, potatoes, peanuts, peas, and green beans.*

Dieters who take chromium picolinate supplements at doses higher than what is recommended are putting themselves at *risk of developing side effects.* These include weight gain caused by binges to satisfy increased cravings, excessive thirst, frequent urination leading to the loss of vital minerals in the body, increased craving for sweets, sleepiness or drowsiness during the day, cold sweats, cold and clammy hands, dizziness, and irritability after going for six hours without food. Keeping this and the relatively high levels of naturally occurring chromium in my meal plan in mind, I recommend that *you get your chromium from your diet.*

A Word about Gluten Intolerance

Celiac disease is different from gluten sensitivity. Celiac disease is a condition that affects one in every 133 people in the United States. It is a serious condition that requires strict adherence to a gluten-free diet. It is detected through a blood test. Until recently, people who got *negative results* on a blood test and intestinal biopsy used to diagnose celiac disease were told to eat whatever they wanted, as gluten was not thought to be causing their health problems. However, many of those people tried a gluten-free diet anyway and reported that they felt much better. Their symptoms, which may have included fatigue, gastrointestinal complaints, and neurological issues, cleared when they ate gluten free.

Now, some researchers are saying that a condition they are calling "gluten sensitivity," "non-celiac gluten sensitivity" (NCGS), "gluten intolerance," or even "gluten allergy" does exist. However, the condition's existence has not yet been proven definitively. There is no scientific explanation for why it occurs and how it might be related to celiac disease.

If you are sensitive to gluten, trying to avoid it may make you feel a lot better. This can be done by trial and error, where you eliminate products containing gluten for two weeks, and then reintroduce products with gluten one at a time, to monitor your reaction. Symptoms such as diarrhea, constipation, bloating, and abdominal pain happen frequently in those who have been diagnosed with gluten sensitivity. Fatigue, joint pain, headaches, and brain fog also are common.

To avoid products with gluten is not easy, but today many food companies will expressly state on the label if a product is gluten free. Since interest in eating gluten free is on the rise, food manufacturers are responding, and now there are many tasty and nutritious options available. Also, try buying *natural, unprocessed foods that are naturally gluten free.* For example, fresh fruit, vegetables, nuts, poultry, meat, and fish do not contain any gluten when they are unprocessed, so you can always buy these items knowing that they are safe to eat.

If you are gluten sensitive, always avoid processed food. The more processed a food is, the greater the chance it contains gluten, because gluten is often used as a protein or a thickening or stabilizing agent. If you are *not* gluten sensitive or do *not* have celiac disease, there is no evidence that eating gluten free will make you feel better or lose weight.

A Word about Organic Produce

Although organic produce can be more costly than conventionally grown foods, it is sometimes a very wise investment to buy organic. It is essential to pay the price of organics for certain produce in particular. *Conventional* agriculture uses pesticides, herbicides, chemical fertilizers, and fungicides to increase its yield of crops. Some of these are highly toxic and even carcinogenic. These chemicals accumulate in your body fat and can cause nerve damage, disrupted fetal brain development, and cancer. Some chemicals can remain in your body for decades. Although you will reduce the amount of chemicals by washing conventionally grown produce, they will not be completely eliminated.

Organic produce is more costly than conventionally grown produce. If you are on a budget (and who isn't?), it is wise to choose to buy organic for the fruits and vegetables that carry the most pesticides.

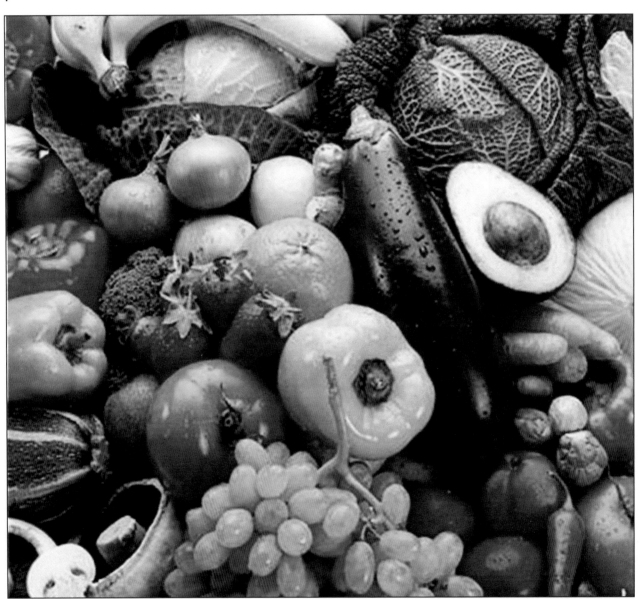

Fruits and vegetables with thin or edible skins tend to get sprayed more and absorb more pesticide residue. **Here is a list of the top ten foods to buy organic:**

1. **Apples**: The skin of apples has lots of vitamins, so you don't want to peel it off. But even if you do, apples are a big pest target, heavily sprayed, and often washing and peeling doesn't get off all of the chemicals.

2. **Blueberries:** These antioxidant powerhouse berries are among the "dirtiest" of fruits. They are sprayed with dozens of pesticides so make sure you buy fresh, organic blueberries.

3. **Grapes:** It is important to buy organic grapes and organic wines. Grapes have thin skin and are sprayed various times during the growing process.

4. **Peaches and Nectarines:** These fruits are heavily sprayed, and their delicate skin absorbs the chemicals easily.

5. **Celery:** Celery is sprayed with organophosphates, which have been linked to ADHD. With no protective skin, they absorb harmful chemicals rapidly that do not wash off.

6. **Bell Peppers:** Bell peppers' soft skin and lack of a protective layer make them an organic must-buy.

7. **Potatoes:** Potatoes are among the most contaminated veggies. If you cannot find organic, opt for sweet potatoes instead.

8. **Spinach:** Spinach is among the most heavily sprayed leafy green, which puts it on the must-buy organic list.

9. **Meat:** Chicken, turkey, and beef store chemicals and hormones in their fat, so buy organic meat. Stay away from fatty cuts and chicken thighs. Also, sometimes switch to organic tofu as a substitution.

10. **Coffee:** Coffee beans grown in other countries are not regulated, so look for the USDA Organic label to ensure your coffee does not come with a shot of harmful chemicals.

Part II

My Recipes

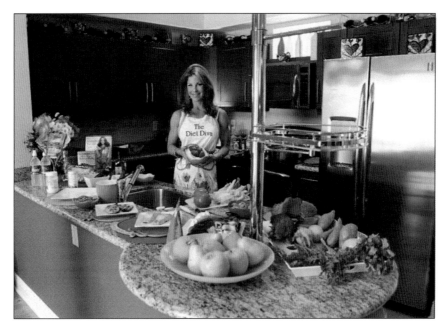

The collection of recipes in this book is meant for you to enjoy while you are on my meal plans. They meet the dietary requirements of fat-blasting, muscle-building fuel. I love to cook healthful, delicious meals for my family and me to enjoy.

Remember, *eating healthy does not equal eating boring, bland, and dry food*. Nor does it equal deprivation. Food should appeal to all the senses and should optimize your health and wellness. Although there are many, many more things I enjoy making, I am only including a few recipes in this book. These are things that my family and I eat a lot of.

Chapter 11: Breakfasts

Healthy Egg-White Omelet

This healthy treat takes just a few minutes to whip together and is loaded with protein and virtually fat free. Enjoy with small bowl of oatmeal or a piece of Ezekiel toast.

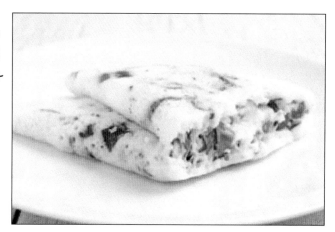

Ingredients

- 1/2 tbsp olive oil
- 1/3 cup chopped onion
- 3 cups chopped spinach
- 1/4 tsp black pepper
- 5 egg whites

Directions

1. Heat olive oil in a nonstick skillet on medium high heat and sauté onions until golden brown.

2. Add spinach to wilt.

3. Whisk egg whites lightly with black pepper and pour on top of vegetables.

4. Cook over medium heat until set. Flip and brown other side.

5. Serve and enjoy.

Nutrients per serving:
110 calories, 2 g fat, 1 g carbohydrates, 19 g protein

Oatmeal

Makes 1 serving

Ingredients

- ¼ cup steel-cut oats
- ¼ cup fat-free milk
- slivered almonds
- ½ cup blueberries
- 1 tsp flaxseed

Studies show that oatmeal prevents heart attack, stroke, and obesity. Start your day off right with this slow-burning complex carbohydrate to enjoy all the benefits.

Directions

1. Boil 1 cup of water over high heat.

2. Add oats. Cook, stirring, for 25 minutes, until the oatmeal is soft.

3. Reduce heat to low and cook for 3 more minutes, stirring constantly.

4. Add milk, almonds, fresh or frozen blueberries, and flaxseed.

5. Mix and serve.

Nutrients per serving:
218 calories, 5.2 g fat, 40 g carbohydrates, 10 g protein

Quick Oatmeal with Protein

This is a recipe I make every day for my sons to get them off to school with full and happy stomachs. It's quick and easy, and they love the flavor. Ingredients

- 1 package instant, no-sugar-added oatmeal
- 1 scoop vanilla protein powder
- ¾ cup water
- 7 chopped walnuts
- ¼ chopped banana

Directions

1. Cook oatmeal as per package instructions.

2. Cool down slightly.

3. Stir in remaining ingredients.

4. Enjoy this protein-rich, super-healthy breakfast!

Nutrients per serving:
258 calories, 5 g fat, 48 g carbohydrate, 23 g protein

Willie's Favorite Breakfast Shake

Enjoy this healthy shake on those mornings when you are rushed for time. It's a complete breakfast in a cup! Willie drinks this every morning for a super-charged way to get his breakfast in a minute.

Ingredients

- ¼ cup oatmeal
- 1 scoop vanilla whey protein powder
- 4 oz. cold water
- ¼ cup liquid egg whites
- ½ cup frozen blueberries
- 4 ice cubes

Directions

1. Pour all ingredients together in a blender.

2. Blend together for a full cycle.

3. Pour into a tall glass and enjoy!

Nutrients per serving:
354 calories, 4 g fat, 38 g carbohydrates, 44 g protein

Quick and Easy Sunday Morning Protein Pancakes

Warning! These pancakes are addicting. My kids love them, and I make them every Sunday morning as a special treat. You can modify the added ingredients to suit your needs and taste buds. My family loves the bananas together with the walnuts and some yummy, unsweetened dark chocolate morsels. Delicious!

Ingredients

- 1 cup whole-wheat pancake mix
- 1 cup oatmeal
- 1 scoop vanilla protein powder
- 2 tbsp coconut oil
- 1 whole egg
- 1 cup nonfat milk
- 1 banana, chopped into bite-sized pieces
- ¼ cup chopped walnuts
- ¼ cup semisweet chocolate chips, if desired

Directions

1. Mix together pancake mix, protein powder, and oatmeal.

2. Add coconut oil, egg, and milk.

3. Stir until large lumps have disappeared.

4. Add the remaining ingredients.

5. Drop into skillet over medium heat by large spoonfuls.

6. Cook until set or golden brown, then flip and cook other side.

Enjoy!

Nutrients per serving:
140 calories, 4 g fat, 21 g carbohydrates, 15 g protein

Breakfast Burritos

Ingredients

- organic vegetable cooking spray
- 4 egg whites
- 1 whole-wheat tortilla
- ¼ cup rinsed canned beans (such as pinto beans or black beans)
- salsa (to taste)

The average egg contains about 6.3 grams of protein, 3.6 of which come from the egg white. In addition to protein, other nutrients found in the egg white are riboflavin, niacin, folate, vitamin B12, calcium, iron, copper, zinc, and sodium. Of the 72 calories in an egg, one white has about 17.

Directions

1. Spray vegetable cooking spray into a frying pan.
2. Scramble the egg whites in the pan and cook to the desired degree of doneness.
3. Place the cooked eggs on the tortillas.
4. Place the beans on top of the eggs.
5. Roll each tortilla into a wrap.
6. Microwave for 30 seconds.
7. Spoon salsa on top.

Nutrients per serving:
220 calories, 3 g fat, 34 g carbohydrates, 10 g protein

Chapter 12: Lunches

Coach Willie's Lean Turkey Burgers

Ingredients

- 1¼ lbs. ground lean turkey
- ½ cup finely shredded carrot
- ½ cup finely diced bell peppers
- ¼ cup finely chopped red onion
- 2 tbsp lemon juice
- 2 tsp sodium free Ms. Dash seasoning
- 2 tsp garlic powder
- ½ tsp black pepper

Ground turkey is a good substitute for ground beef or pork. Turkey is a leaner meat, and it contains less fat. Instead of frying the turkey burger in oil on the stove top, you can bake it in the oven.

Directions

1. In a bowl, mix turkey, vegetables, and all seasonings together.

2. Let sit for at least half an hour.

3. Separate into patties.

4. Preheat oven to 375 degrees.

5. Bake for 15 minutes; then turn over and bake an additional 10 minutes or until burgers are cooked through but still juicy. The burgers should reach an internal temperature of 165 degrees.

Nutrients per serving:
188 calories, 6 g fat, 2.7 g carbohydrates, 23 g protein

Oriental Chicken Salad

Makes 6 servings

Ingredients

- 1 recipe Asian Salad Dressing (below)
- ¼ cup fresh cilantro, minced
- 2 tbsp fresh ginger, grated or minced
- 10 oz. fresh baby spinach, arugula, or other salad greens mix
- 2 cups sliced bell peppers, red, yellow, or orange
- 3 green onions, thinly sliced
- 3 chicken breasts, grilled and chopped
- ½–1 cup roasted, unsalted peanuts, crushed
- ½ mango, pitted, peeled, and diced

Directions

1. Mix dressing, cilantro, and ginger in a small bowl. Let stand.

2. Toss salad greens with peppers, onions, chicken, and peanuts. Dress salad to taste and toss to combine.

3. Add mango and serve.

Asian Salad Dressing

- 3 tbsp rice wine vinegar
- 1 tbsp lime juice
- 3 tbsp low-sodium soy sauce
- ½ tsp dry mustard
- 2 tsp sesame oil
- ¼ cup peanut oil or other mild salad oil

Nutrients per serving:
228 calories, 4 g fat, 20 g carbohydrates, 28 g protein

Unni's Favorite Easy Ceviche

I love having this great meal on hand, and I make it all the time. The fresh lime juice really makes a difference. And you can't get a much cleaner protein meal than this. This dish can be stored covered in the fridge for three to four days and enjoyed with a large green salad as a super-healthy meal.

Ingredients

- 2 lbs. tilapia or other firm white fish fillets, finely cubed
- 8–10 garlic cloves, chopped
- ½ tsp black pepper
- 2 tsp fresh cilantro, chopped
- 1 habanero pepper, seeded and chopped
- 8–12 limes, freshly squeezed and strained to remove pulp, enough to completely cover fish
- 1 red onion, thinly sliced and rinsed

Directions

1. Combine all ingredients except red onion and mix well.

2. Put into serving dish.

3. Cover with red onions and chill in fridge for at least two hours.

Nutrients per serving:
198 calories, 2.8 g fat, 12 g carbohydrates, 31 g protein

Chicken Lettuce Bowls

You can use a slow cooker for this tasty recipe.

Ingredients

- 1 lb. chicken breast, cut into 1" pieces
- 1½ cups dry wild rice mix
- 2¾ cups low-sodium vegetable broth
- 1 shallot, finely chopped
- 1 medium carrot, peeled and finely chopped
- 1 celery rib, finely chopped
- 8 oz. sugar snap peas, trimmed and halved
- 2 tbsp raspberry vinegar
- ½ cup toasted walnuts chopped
- ¼ cup chopped parsley
- ½ tsp sea salt
- ¼ tsp black pepper
- 1 large head Boston Bibb lettuce

Directions

1. Rinse and drain rice. Place rice in slow cooker and add broth, chicken, shallots, carrots, and celery.

2. Cover and cook on low for 5 hours or until rice is ready but not mushy.

3. Stir in sugar snap peas, vinegar, walnuts, parsley, and salt.

4. Spoon about ½ cup of rice mixture into the bowl-shaped, cleaned leaves of the lettuce head.

5. Serve.

Nutrients per serving:
127 calories, 3 g fat, 5 g carbohydrates, 19 g protein

Healthy Veggie and Shrimp Frittata

This is another one of our staples that can be made ahead and enjoyed for dinner or even the next day as yummy leftovers.

Ingredients

- ½ cup diced onion
- 1–2 cloves minced garlic
- ½ cup sliced fresh mushrooms
- 1 cup chopped bell pepper
- 1 cup quartered artichoke hearts, rinsed and drained
- 2 whole eggs
- 1½ cup liquid egg whites
- organic cooking vegetable oil spray
- 12 large cooked shrimp
- Ms. Dash seasoning

Directions

1. Heat oil in a large skillet over medium heat; cook and stir mushrooms, green onion, and bell pepper until tender, about 5 minutes.

2. Stir in diced tomato and egg mixture; as eggs set, lift edges, letting uncooked portion flow underneath. Cook until egg mixture sets, 10 to 15 minutes.

3. Cut into wedges and serve immediately.

Nutrients per serving:
190 calories, 4.1 g fat, 12 g carbohydrates, 23 g protein

Veggie Mushroom Burgers

Ingredients

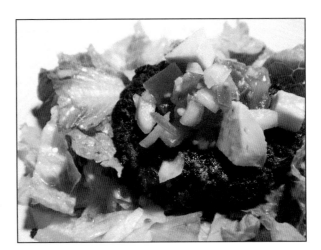

- 1/3 cup wheat flour
- ¼ chopped onion
- 2 cups chopped mushrooms
- 1/3 cup wheat bran
- ½ tsp baking powder
- 4 egg whites
- garlic, Ms. Dash Italian spice, and basil to taste

Directions

1. Combine all the ingredients in a large bowl.

2. Make into four patties and brown in a nonstick skillet over medium-high heat until heated or approximately 4 minutes on each side.

3. Serve with a large green salad.

Nutrients per serving:
130 calories, 1.1 g fat, 26.3 g carbohydrate, 11 g protein

Chapter 13: Dinners

"Diet Diva" Oven-Baked Tilapia

Serves 4

Serve this easy and tasty baked tilapia dish with brown rice, quinoa, or baked sweet potatoes.

Ingredients

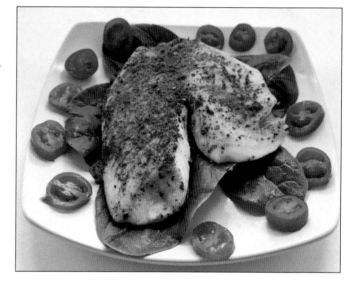

- 4–6 tilapia filets
- organic, silicone-free cooking spray
- 8–12 oz. baby spinach, cleaned
- ¼ teaspoon onion powder
- 1–2 tbsp lemon juice
- Ms. Dash Caribbean seasoning blend to taste
- 1 tomato, chopped
- 4 green onions, thinly sliced

Directions

1. Spray a 9x13-inch baking dish with cooking spray and add the spinach. If necessary to make the spinach fit it into the baking dish, steam or sauté it for a minute or two to wilt slightly.

2. Sprinkle spinach with pepper and onion powder. Sprinkle tilapia filets lightly with seasonings. Arrange the filets over the spinach and sprinkle with chopped tomato and sliced green onion.

3. Cover baking dish with foil and bake at 350° for 20 to 25 minutes or until fish flakes easily with a fork.

Nutrients per serving:
137 calories, 2.5 g fat, 4.7 g carbohydrates, 25 g protein

Shrimp Quinoa

Ingredients

- ½ cup uncooked quinoa, rinsed
- ¾ cup chicken broth
- olive oil spray
- 1½ cloves garlic, minced
- ½ onion, diced
- ½ red bell pepper, diced
- 4 spears fresh asparagus, trimmed and cut into 1-inch pieces
- ½ cup sliced fresh mushrooms
- 1½ tsp minced fresh ginger root
- ½ lb. uncooked medium shrimp, peeled and deveined
- 1½ tsp lemon juice
- pepper to taste

Directions

1. Bring the quinoa and chicken broth to a boil in a saucepan over high heat. Reduce heat to medium low, cover, and simmer until the quinoa is tender, about 15 minutes. Turn off the heat, and let the remaining liquid absorb into the quinoa.

2. Meanwhile, heat the olive oil in a large skillet over medium heat. Stir in the garlic, onion, and red bell pepper; cook and stir until the onion has softened and turned translucent, about 5 minutes. Add the asparagus, mushrooms, and ginger; continue cooking until the asparagus is tender. Stir in the shrimp and cook until the shrimp have turned pink and are no longer translucent in the center.

3. Stir the lemon juice into the quinoa, and then toss the quinoa with the shrimp and vegetable mixture. Season with pepper before serving.

Nutrients per serving:
267 calories, 3 g fat, 37 g carbohydrates, 23 g protein

Ginger Halibut

Ingredients

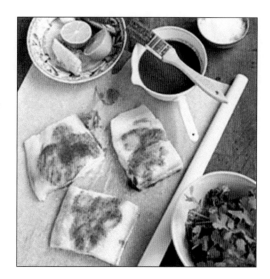

- 1 clove garlic, peeled
- ½ small jalapeno pepper
- 1 piece fresh ginger (½ inch), peeled and roughly chopped
- 3 tbsp freshly squeezed lime juice (2 limes)
- 1 cup loosely packed cilantro leaves
- 4 tbsp olive oil
- salt and freshly ground black pepper
- 1 halibut fillet (1½ lbs.), skin removed and cut into equal pieces

Directions

1. Combine garlic, jalapeno, ginger, lime juice, and cilantro in the jar of a blender. Cover blender and remove the stopper. Turn on blender and slowly drizzle in the olive oil. Process until mixture is bright green and smooth. Season cilantro sauce to taste with salt and black pepper.

2. Season both sides of fillets with salt and black pepper. Brush the top of each fillet with 1 tablespoon cilantro sauce.

3. Fill a large high-sided skillet with 1 inch water. Set over high heat and bring to a boil. Set a steamer basket in the skillet, and arrange fillets in basket. Cover and steam until fish has just cooked through but is still moist, 5 to 6 minutes. Remove fish from steamer, drizzle with additional cilantro sauce, and serve.

Nutrients per serving:
264 calories, 4 g fat, 4.5 g carbohydrate, 27 g protein

Coconut Lime Chicken

Ingredients

- 5 oz. chicken breast
- 1 tbsp coconut flour
- 1 tbsp shredded unsweetened coconut
- 1 tsp coconut oil
- juice of ½ lime

Directions

1. Cut chicken breast into chunks and place in a mixing bowl with coconut flour and shredded coconut. Toss together to coat.

2. Heat a skillet over medium-high heat. Coat the pan with coconut oil. Spread the coated chicken evenly over the pan and brown for 3 to 4 minutes per side. Squeeze the lime juice over the chicken and cook another 1 to 2 minutes.

3. Serve with brown rice or inside Bibb lettuce bowls. Garnish with red pepper slices.

Nutrients per serving:
300 calories, 12 g fat, 12 g carbohydrates, 35 g protein

Cashew Chicken with Water Chestnuts

Ingredients

- 1/3 cup low-sodium vegetable broth
- 1 tbsp and 1½ tsp soy sauce
- ¼ tsp ground ginger
- ¼ tsp hot pepper sauce
- 1 tbsp coconut oil
- ½ lb. skinless, boneless chicken breast meat, cut into strips
- ½ small onion, chopped
- ½ green bell pepper, chopped
- ½ 8-oz. can sliced water chestnuts, drained
- 1/3 cup cashews

Directions

1. To make the sauce: Add vegetable broth to a medium pan, and stir in the soy sauce, ginger, and hot sauce; set aside. Heat half of the coconut oil in a wok or large skillet over high heat. Stir in the chicken; cook and stir until the chicken is no longer pink, about 5 minutes. Remove the chicken from the wok, and set aside.

2. Pour the remaining amount of coconut oil into the wok, and stir in the onion, green bell pepper, and water chestnuts. Cook and stir until the chestnuts are hot and the onion has softened, about 5 minutes more. Stir up the sauce, then pour into the wok, and bring to a boil. Add the reserved chicken, and stir until the sauce thickens, and the chicken is hot. Sprinkle with cashews to serve.

Nutrients per serving:
364 calories, 18 g fat, 15 g carbohydrate, 27 g protein

Black Bean Burger

This is another recipe for my vegetarian or vegan friends or those days when you just want to eliminate meat. As these are slightly higher in carbohydrates than animal-source protein, prepare and eat them with a large green salad. You can also eat them on days that require glycogen loading, such as the day before you work out legs. The best part is that these burgers are ready in only fifteen minutes.

Makes 1 serving

Ingredients

- ½ cup rinsed black beans
- ¼ cup whole-wheat flour
- ½ cup shredded carrots
- 1 egg white
- ¼ tsp cumin
- ¼ tsp freshly ground pepper
- 1 whole-wheat bun
- 1 tbsp salsa
- arugula, to garnish
- olive oil cooking spray

Directions

1. In a mixing bowl, mash beans, flour, cumin, pepper, and egg white together. Add carrots and press into a patty.

2. Heat skillet over medium to high heat and coat lightly with cooking spray. Cook patty for 3 minutes on each side.

3. Place arugula and patty on bun and top with salsa.

Nutrients per serving:
370 calories, 2 g fat, 69 g carbohydrate, 18 g protein

Braised Balsamic Chicken

Serves 2

Ingredients

- 2 skinless, preferably organic, boneless chicken breast halves
- ground black pepper to taste
- ¼ tsp chopped garlic
- 2 tsp olive oil
- 3/8 onion, thinly sliced
- 2 tbsp balsamic vinegar
- 1 1/2 cup low-sodium diced tomatoes
- ¼ tsp dried basil
- ¼ tsp dried oregano
- ¼ tsp dried rosemary
- 1/8 tsp dried thyme

Directions

1. Season chicken breasts with ground black pepper and garlic. Heat olive oil in a medium skillet, and brown the onion and seasoned chicken breasts.

2. Pour tomatoes and balsamic vinegar over chicken, and then season with basil, oregano, rosemary and thyme. Simmer until chicken is no longer pink and the juices run clear, about 15 minutes.

3. Serve with steamed green beans and brown rice.

Nutrients per serving:
270 calories, 5 g fat, 8 g carbohydrate, 28 g protein

Teriyaki Salmon with Zucchini

Ingredients

- 5 tbsp low-sodium teriyaki sauce or liquid Braggs Amino Acids
- 2 6-oz. salmon fillets
- sesame seeds
- 2 small zucchini, thinly sliced
- 4 scallions, chopped
- cooking spray

Directions

1. Combine teriyaki sauce or Bragg's Aminos and fish in a ziplock plastic bag. Seal and marinate 20 minutes.

2. Toast sesame seeds in a large, nonstick skillet over medium heat, and set aside.

3. Drain fish, discarding marinade.

4. Add fish to skillet and cook 5 minutes. Turn and cook for 5 more minutes over medium-low heat.

5. Remove from skillet and keep warm.

6. Add the zucchini, scallions, and cooking spray to skillet.

7. Sauté 4 minutes or until lightly browned.

8. Sprinkle with sesame seeds and serve.

Nutrients per serving:
288 calories, 12 g fat, 7 g carbohydrate, 38 g protein

Quinoa Jambalaya

Ingredients

- 1 tbsp canola oil
- ½ onion, chopped
- 1 zucchini, chopped
- 1 red bell pepper, chopped
- 1 garlic clove, minced
- 1 low-sodium, all-natural chicken sausage, sliced into 6 rounds (try Applegate Farms)
- ¼ cup dry quinoa
- ½ cup low-sodium vegetable broth
- 1 can fire-roasted tomatoes
- ¼ lb. shrimp, peeled and deveined
- sea salt and pepper, to taste
- 1 green onion, sliced thinly

Quinoa is an excellent source of protien. In face, it is the only grain that is a complete protein, containing all the amino acids.

Directions

1. Heat oil in a large, nonstick skillet over medium-high heat. Sauté onion, zucchini, bell pepper, garlic, and sausage slices for 5 minutes. Add the quinoa and toss to coat, about 2 minutes.

2. Add broth and tomatoes to skillet and bring to a boil. Then reduce heat and simmer, covered, for 10 minutes.

3. Add the shrimp and cover the pan. Cook an additional 5 to 10 minutes, or until the shrimp are opaque and cooked through.

4. Add salt and pepper to taste. Remove from heat and place onto plates. Top with green onions. Serve.

Nutrients per serving:
389 calories, 15 g fat, 39 g carbohydrates, 24 g protein

Grilled Salmon with Pineapple Salsa

Ingredients

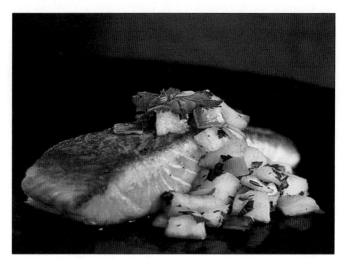

- 1 cup chopped fresh pineapple

- 2 tbsp finely chopped red onion

- 2 tbsp chopped cilantro

- 1 tbsp rice vinegar

- 1/8 tsp ground red pepper

- cooking spray

- 4 6-oz. salmon fillets (about ½-inch thick)

Directions

1. Combine first five ingredients (through pepper) in a bowl; set aside.

2. Heat a nonstick grill pan coated with cooking spray over medium-high heat. Sprinkle fish with salt. Cook fish 4 minutes on each side or until it flakes easily when tested with a fork. Top with salsa.

Nutrients per serving:
294 calories, 13 g fat, 5.6 g carbohydrates, 36 g protein

Chapter 14: Spice It Up

Eating right does not have to mean boring, bland food. Make your meals flavorful and enjoyable by adding some "spice" that is healthy and low calorie.

Fresh Tomato Salsa

Ingredients

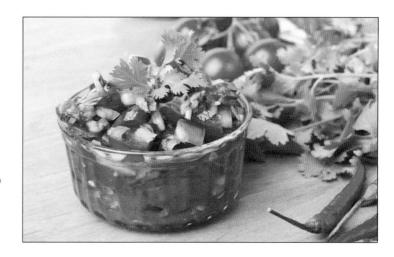

- 3 tomatoes, finely chopped
- ½ cup finely diced onion
- 5 serrano chilies, finely chopped
- ½ cup chopped fresh cilantro
- 1 tsp salt
- 2 tsp lime juice

Directions

1. In a medium bowl, stir together tomatoes, onion, chili peppers, cilantro, salt, and lime juice.

2. Chill for one hour in the refrigerator before serving.

Nutrients per serving:
51 calories, 0.2 g fat, 5 g carbohydrates, 1 g protein

Mango, Jicama, and Black Bean Salsa

A great South Florida treat, this salsa is delicious and nutritious and gives a distinct tropical flavor to many of your dishes.

Ingredients

- 1½ cups diced fresh mango
- ¾ cup diced jicama
- ¾ cup cooked black beans, drained
- 1 tsp finely chopped jalapeno
- 2 tsp finely chopped fresh mint
- 1/3 cup finely chopped red onion
- 2 tsp fresh lime juice
- 2 tsp rice vinegar
- ½ tsp salt

Mango is high in vitamin A and has been found to protect against certain cancers due to high antioxidant content.

Directions

1. In a food processor or blender, purée ½ cup of the diced mango until smooth.

2. In a serving bowl, combine the remaining diced mango, jicama, beans, jalapeno, mint, onion, lime juice, and vinegar.

3. Gently stir in the mango purée. Season with salt.

4. Let stand for 20 minutes before serving.

Nutrients per serving (2 tbsp):
19 calories, 0 g fat, 4 g carbohydrate, 1 g protein

The Diet Diva's Favorite Ratatouille

This is another one of my staple dishes that can be made ahead, stored, and reheated and enjoyed for days. I top almost everything with this delicious and nutrient-dense vegetable stew.

Ingredients

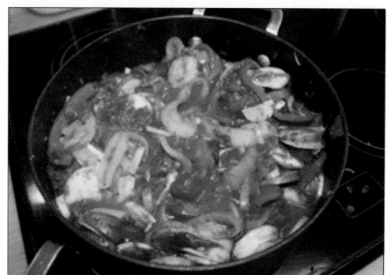

- 3 tbsp extra-virgin olive oil
- 1 large eggplant (about 1 lb.), trimmed and sliced or diced
- 1 medium onion, sliced or diced
- 2 medium zucchini (1 lb. total), trimmed and sliced or diced
- 2 cloves garlic, minced
- 1 14.5-ounce can or box no-salt-added diced tomatoes,
- 1 can organic tomato paste
- 1 tsp Ms. Dash Italian salt-free seasoning, or ½ tsp dried thyme mixed with ¼ tsp each dried rosemary and dried marjoram
- ½ tsp freshly ground black pepper
- ¼ cup chopped fresh or dried basil

Directions

1. In a large, nonstick skillet, heat 1 tablespoon of the olive oil over medium-high heat. Add the eggplant and cook, stirring, until it has softened but not completely lost its shape, about 5 minutes. Remove the eggplant from the skillet.

2. Heat another tablespoon of oil in the same skillet over medium-high heat. Add the onion and cook, stirring, until softened and translucent, about 5 minutes. Add the zucchini and garlic to the pan and cook, stirring occasionally, until the zucchini is softened, 6 to 7 minutes.

3. Return the eggplant to pan and add the tomatoes and seasonings. Simmer for approximately 20 minutes. Stir in the basil and remaining tablespoon oil.

Nutrients per serving:
180 calories, 8g fat, 18 g carbohydrate, 4 g protein

Chapter 15: Snacks

Cucumber Carrot Salad

Serves 2

Ingredients

- ½ cucumber, sliced
- ½ 8-oz. package baby carrots
- ½ lime, juiced
- ½ tsp chili powder
- 1/8 tsp salt
- pinch cayenne pepper, or more to taste (optional)

Directions

Combine the cucumber, baby carrots, lime juice, chili powder, salt, and cayenne pepper in a bowl; toss to combine evenly.

Nutrients per serving:
34 calories, 0 g fat, 6 g carbohydrate, 1 g protein

Peanut Butter Banana Roll-Ups

Ingredients

- 1 ripe banana
- 1½ tbsp peanut butter
- 1 whole-wheat tortilla-style flatbread
- ½ tbsp chia seeds

Directions

1. Spread tortilla with peanut butter.

2. Place banana on the one side of the tortilla and sprinkle with chia seeds.

3. Roll tortilla and banana until the banana is completely wrapped in the tortilla. Enjoy!

Nutrients per serving:

280 calories, 12 g fat, 36 g carbohydrate, 18 g protein

Chocolate Protein Treats

This is a nontraditional treat, but it serves the purpose of some sweetness combined with health for me. Try it if you feel adventurous.

Ingredients

- 1 cup Fage unsweetened vanilla Greek yogurt
- 1 scoop vanilla protein powder
- 1 cup oats
- 2 tbsp unsweetened cocoa powder
- 1 tsp liquid Stevia vanilla extract

Chia seeds are high in fiber, which helps stabilize blood sugar and keep you fuller longer.

Directions

1. Combine all ingredients.

2. Stir until blended and smooth in texture.

3. Put into 4 small individual serving cups.

4. Chill in refrigerator for ½ hour.

5. Enjoy.

Nutrients per serving:

80 calories, 2 g fat, 6 g carbohydrate, 20 g protein

Chapter 16: How to Prepare Healthy Fish Dishes

Many of the meal options in these plans feature fish dishes. Fish is a low-calorie, high-protein, nutrient-dense food. Here are some tips on how to prepare this wonderful staple.

Grilled Fish

When you're grilling fish, keep a close watch. Fish only takes a few minutes per side to cook. If the fillets are an even thickness, sometimes they don't even require flipping and can be cooked through by grilling on one side only.

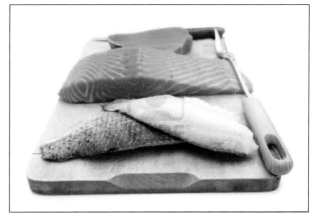

- Brush the fish lightly with oil or spray with organic, nonstick cooking spray.

- Place fish near the edge of the grill, away from the hottest part of the fire. (Don't try to lift up the fish right away; it will be stuck to the grill.)

- Start checking for color and doneness after a few minutes, once the fish starts to release some of its juices.

- Flip the fish over when you see light grill marks forming.

Steamed Fish

Steaming is another gentle cooking method. It produces a mild-tasting fish that is free of oils or added fat.

- Rub the fish with spices, chopped herbs, ginger, garlic, and chili peppers to infuse flavor while it cooks.
- Use a bamboo steamer or a folding steamer basket with enough room for each piece of fish to lie flat.
- Pour about one-and-a-half inches of water into the pan.
- Place the steamer over the water, cover the pot, and bring the water to a boil.
- Begin checking the fish for doneness after ten minutes.

Broiled Fish

When the weather's not right for grilling, try broiling instead. Broiling is great when you want a fast, simple, hassle-free preparation with delicious results. It gives fish a nicely browned exterior with the convenience of a temperature-controlled heat source.Preheat oven to broil setting.

- Brush the fish lightly with oil or spray with organic nonstick cooking spray.
- Place fish near the top of the oven.
- Start checking for color and doneness after a few minutes, once the fish starts to release some of its juices.
- For easy cleanup, line the broiler pan with a piece of foil.

Poached Fish

This gentle cooking method is perfect for seafood. Poaching keeps fish moist and won't mask the delicate flavor. To poach fish, use vegetable broth or just plain water. Use a pan big enough to lay each piece of fish down flat.

- Pour in enough liquid to just barely cover the fish.
- Bring the liquid to a simmer and keep it there.
- If you see any bubbles coming up from the bottom of the pan, it's too hot. The liquid should be at a simmer. The ideal poaching temperature is between 165 and 180 degrees Fahrenheit.
- When fish changes to solid color or gets firm, it is done.

Part III

The Meal Plans

And now, you are ready to get on the best eating plan to blast fat, gain lean muscle, reduce hunger pangs and cravings, stoke your metabolism and get hot and healthy.

Chapter 17: The Diet Diva 1,500-Calorie, Twenty-Eight-Day Fat-Blasting Meal Plan

This is the plan to be on for *steady fat loss*, while *keeping or even increasing* your hard-earned muscle. Make sure to eat all your meals and drink at least eight full glasses of water per day. You may also drink black coffee, tea, or seltzer water, as much as you wish. Make sure to use Truvia or Stevia to sweeten, and skip the sugar completely. Your food should be seasoned with salt-free seasonings. Also, you should consider taking a multivitamin daily. As always, before starting any diet or exercise regimen, make sure to consult with a licensed physician first.

To season your food daily, you may use cilantro, fresh salsa, cinnamon, pepper, garlic, lemon or lemon juice, balsamic vinegar, and a small amount of olive oil or coconut oil. You can also use the nonstick vegetable spray for cooking.

All meals range between 1,400 and 1,600 calories per day. This is a good daily caloric intake for a 130-to-140-pound person on a one-to-two-pounds-of-fat-loss-per-week meal plan, assuming that you are doing regular, sustained physical activity in conjunction with the eating plan. If you are heavier and need to consume more food, try the same plan, but add a bit more lean protein and complex carbs per day.

Please enjoy plenty of water while you are on this plan. Not only are you losing water while working out, but you need it to speed up fat loss and increase the removal of waste products and metabolize protein as well.

It is very *important that you eat your snacks each day.* Not only does this ensure that your metabolism stays fueled up, but it also prevents you from getting too hungry in the evening and then possibly overeating. Remember: you must eat more to lose more.

Your first meal should be breakfast, and it should be eaten within thirty minutes of waking up. Thereafter it is *very important that each meal/snack be spaced at three-hour intervals.* In fact, as you progress into the meal plan and your metabolism fires up, you may notice that you get hungry even more often. *Do not wait out hunger pangs!* Instead, keep your metabolism burning, by adding a *small* snack such as a protein shake or ten raw almonds. If you do not want to add additional snacks, opt to space your meals at two-and-a-half-hour intervals instead. In the evening, if you are hungry before going to bed, you may add the small snack we just talked about, or you can even opt to have a low-sugar popsicle (such as Weight Watchers brand), sugar-free Jell-O, hot herbal tea, or some raw veggies with one tablespoon of nut butter.

If, for instance, you eat breakfast at seven a.m., your midmorning snack is at ten a.m., your lunch at one p.m., your late afternoon snack is at four p.m., and your dinner at seven p.m. Eating every three hours ensures that your metabolism stays *fired up. Eat by the clock, not by your stomach or your hunger level.*

As you progress into this eating plan, you will notice that your body will respond to getting fueled up every three hours by burning more and losing more fat. You will be hungry after three hours, but that's OK, because it means your body burned right through what you ate and is now ready for more of the high-quality, nutrient-packed fuel that you provide it.

While on this meal plan, you will eat simple, unprocessed foods. Stay away from processed and fried foods, anything white, anything with heavy or creamy sauces, and any and all heavy dairy foods.

It is also very important that you *keep the portion sizes as stated* in the meal plan. If you are unsure, please start out by measuring or weighing your food. You will quickly get a hang of the size that your portions should be, thereby ensuring your success.

While I suggest a *protein shake or snack alternative* made with a high-quality, low-sugar protein powder for your midmorning and/or your midafternoon snack, you can make certain substitutions such as the following:

Suggested Snack List

- celery or carrot sticks with 2 tablespoons peanut or almond butter
- 1 high-quality, low-sugar protein bar
- 1 small handful of high-quality, unsalted, natural nuts, such as almonds, walnuts, or pistachios.
- 1 low-fat cheese stick with 5–7 whole-wheat, low-sodium crackers
- 1 hard-boiled egg and 1 cup of raw veggies
- 5–7 crackers with 2 tablespoons hummus
- 2 low-sodium rice cakes with 1 tablespoons almond butter
- ½ cup nonfat yogurt with 3 tablespoons wheat germ or ½ cup low-sugar, high-protein cereal

You get the picture!

The meals on this plan are combined to average about 1,400 to 1,500 calories per day and provide approximately 140 to 150 grams of protein, 100 to 120 grams of carbohydrate, and 50 grams of fat each day. This is the ideal macronutrient breakdown for steady *fat loss*. I have found that consuming 1,500 calories combined with exercise that burns about 250 calories per day leads to a weight loss of one to two pounds of fat per week. *If you feel that you can do with less food or you want a "jump start," please skip ahead to the Diet Diva 1,200-Calorie Seven-Day Metabolism Igniter Meal Plan in the next chapter.*

I have divided the meals as close as possible into a nutritional breakdown as follows:

Breakfast:	Snack:	Lunch:	Snack:	Dinner:	Daily Total:
Carbs: 60 g	3–5 g	15 g	3–5 g	15–30 g	100–120 g
Protein: 30 g	20 g	40 g	20 g	40 g	140–150 g
Fat: 10 g	2–3 g	15 g	2–3 g	20 g	50 g
Calories: 400	150	350	200	400	1,400–1,500 g

The Meal Plan

Day One

Breakfast

Eggs and Turkey

- 3 egg whites
- 2 oz. turkey
- ½ cup berries
- 1 cup cooked oatmeal

Snack

Protein shake or snack alternative

Lunch

Tuna Pita

- 4 oz. low-sodium, water-packed tuna
- 1 whole-wheat pita
- 1 cup cucumber and tomato slices
- 1 cup salad greens
- 1 tsp each olive oil and balsamic vinegar

Snack

Protein shake or snack alternative

Dinner

Chicken with Vegetables

- 4 oz. grilled, skinless chicken, no skin
- 1 small sweet potato
- 1 cup asparagus
- 2 cups salad greens with 1 tsp low-fat dressing

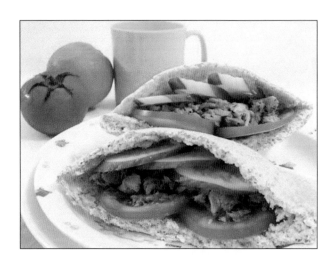

Day Two

Breakfast

Power Up

- 3 egg whites, scrambled
- ½ cup low-fat cottage cheese
- 1 slice Ezekiel bread
- ½ grapefruit

Snack

Protein shake or snack alternative

Lunch

Chicken Pita

- 1 small whole-wheat pita pocket
- 2 tsp hummus
- 1 cup shredded carrot and celery
- 4 oz. low-sodium chicken breast

Snack

Protein shake or snack alternative

Dinner

Teriyaki Salmon

- 4 oz. grilled salmon
- 1 cup sautéed zucchini
- 2 tbsp low-sodium teriyaki sauce
- sesame seeds
- 2 scallions
- 2 tsp canola oil

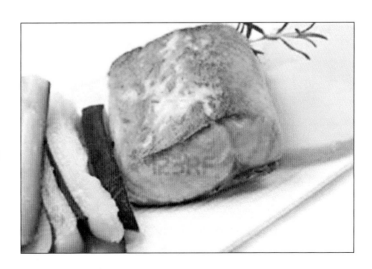

Day Three

Breakfast

Waffle with Cottage Cheese

- 1 whole-grain waffle, such as Van's
- ½ cup cottage cheese
- 6 almonds, chopped
- ½ cup strawberries

Snack

Protein shake or snack alternative

Lunch

Turkey Sandwich

- 4 oz. low-sodium turkey
- 2 slices whole-grain bread, such as Ezekiel
- 1 tsp mustard
- lettuce, tomato slices
- 1 cup low-sodium tomato soup

Snack

Protein shake or snack alternative

Dinner

Baked Cod

- 4 oz. baked cod
- 1 cup steamed broccoli
- ½ cup quinoa cooked in water
- 2 cups salad greens with 1 tsp low-fat dressing

Day Four

Breakfast

Bagel with Peanut Butter

- 1 small whole-grain bagel
- 2 tbsp all-natural peanut butter
- 1 cup cubed cantaloupe
- 9 almonds

Snack

Protein shake or snack alternative

Lunch

Salad with Turkey

- 4 oz. lean, grilled turkey
- 3 cups lettuce
- ¼ cup cherry tomatoes
- ¼ cup slices cucumber
- 1 tbsp low-fat dressing

Snack

Protein shake or snack alternative

Dinner

Baked Cod

- 4 oz. baked cod
- 2 cups mixed green beans, broccoli, and asparagus
- ½ cup brown rice
- 1 tsp olive oil

Day Five

Breakfast

Granola with Yogurt

- ¼ cup low-sugar granola
- 1 cup plain Greek yogurt, such as Fage
- 1 cup mixed berries
- 9 almonds, chopped

Snack

Protein shake or snack alternative

Lunch

Salmon Salad

- 4 oz. grilled or baked salmon
- 2 cups baby spinach
- tomato, bell pepper, mushrooms
- 1 tbsp low-fat dressing
-

Salmon is rich in omega-3 fatty acids, which help brain function and heart health

Snack

Protein shake or snack alternative

Dinner

Chicken Pasta

- 4 oz. grilled chicken breast
- 1 cup cooked whole-wheat pasta
- ½ cup low-sugar tomato sauce
- 1 cup steamed broccoli
- 1 tsp olive oil or low-fat dressing

Day Six

Breakfast

Yogurt and Berries

- 1 cup plain Greek yogurt, such as Fage
- ½ cup high-fiber cereal
- 1 cup mixed berries
- 9 walnuts

Snack

Protein shake or snack alternative

Lunch

Turkey Wrap

- 4 oz. grilled turkey
- 1 whole-wheat tortilla
- 1 cup mixed greens
- ¼ sliced avocado
- 1 tbsp balsamic vinaigrette

Snack

Protein shake or snack alternative

Dinner

Shrimp Quinoa

- 4 oz. sautéed shrimp
- garlic and onion to taste
- 1 cup steamed asparagus
- ½ cup cooked quinoa
- sautéed scallions and green bell peppers for garnish

Day Seven

Breakfast

Whole-Wheat French Toast

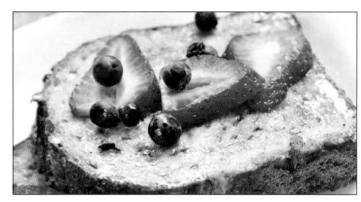

- 1 slice whole-wheat toast soaked in 1 beaten egg
- 1/2 cup low-fat milk
- 1 cup berries
- ½ cup cottage cheese

Combine the milk and the egg, whisk together. Dip your bread into the mix until completely covered. Cook your toast over medium high heat, in a skillet sprayed with cooking oil. Enjoy your French toast garnished with the cottage cheese and the berries.

Snack

Protein shake or snack alternative

Lunch

Shrimp and Pasta

- ½ cup whole-wheat pasta
- 10 steamed asparagus spears
- 4 oz. boiled shrimp
- ½ cup low-sugar marinara sauce *or* 2 tbsp pesto sauce

Snack

Protein shake or snack alternative

Dinner

Oriental Chicken Salad

- 4 oz. grilled chicken
- 12 peanuts
- bell pepper strips, cilantro, baby spinach, green onion, and mango tossed in low-fat ginger dressing

Day Eight

Breakfast

Waffle with Peanut Butter

- 1 whole-grain frozen waffle, such as Van's
- 2 tbsp natural peanut butter
- 1 cup low-fat cottage cheese
- 1 cup cut-up apple

Snack

Protein shake or snack alternative

Lunch

Mediterranean Open-Faced Sandwich

- 1 slice whole-grain bread, such as Ezekiel
- 3 tbsp hummus
- sliced red pepper
- 2 medium slices tomato
- lettuce
- 4 slices low-sodium turkey breast

Snack

Protein shake or snack alternative

Dinner

Chicken with Greens

- 4 oz. broiled, skinless chicken breast
- 1 cup steamed broccoli
- 2 cups mixed greens with 1 tbsp low-fat balsamic dressing

Day Nine

Breakfast

Egg Muffin

- ½ whole-wheat English muffin
- 2 scrambled egg whites
- 2 large tomato slices
- ½ cup low-fat cottage cheese
- 1/8 avocado
- chopped tomato**Snack**

Protein shake or snack alternative

Lunch

Soup and Salad

- 1 cup low-sodium tomato soup
- 2 cups baby spinach
- ½ cup sliced strawberries
- 3 oz. grilled chicken, cubed
- 2 tsp low-fat dressing

Snack

Protein shake or snack alternative

Dinner

Baked Fish and Veggies

- 4 oz. tilapia
- 2 cups mixed green vegetables
- ½ cup chopped canned tomatoes
- 4 oz. baked sweet potato
- 2 tsp vinaigrette

Day Ten

Breakfast

Veggie Omelet

- 1 whole egg and 2 egg whites
- cooking spray
- 1 cup spinach, ½ chopped tomato, and 1 cup chopped mushrooms
- seasoning
- 1 slice whole-wheat toast, such as Ezekiel
- 1 cup skim milk

Snack

Protein shake or snack alternative

Lunch

Chicken Tortilla

- 1 whole-wheat tortilla
- 4 oz. grilled chicken
- chopped bell peppers, artichoke hearts, and tomatoes
- 1 tbsp low-fat dressing or fresh salsa to taste
- carrot and celery sticks on the side

Snack

Protein shake or snack alternative

Dinner

Beef and Green Beans

- 4 oz. beef tenderloin
- steamed cauliflower
- steamed green beans
- small side salad with low-fat dressing

Day Eleven

Breakfast

Oatmeal with Nuts and Blueberries

- ½ cup oatmeal cooked with water and topped with slivered almonds, ½ cup blueberries, and dash cinnamon
- 3 egg whites, scrambled

Snack

Protein shake or snack alternative

Lunch

Shrimp and Pasta

- 7 medium shrimp, sautéed in cooking spray
- ½ cup whole-wheat pasta
- 2 tsp olive oil
- 2 cups steamed broccoli
- ¼ cup cherry tomatoes

Snack

Protein shake or snack alternative

Dinner

Chicken with Vegetables

- 4 oz. broiled, skinless chicken breast
- steamed broccoli
- 2 cups mixed greens with 1 tbsp low-fat balsamic dressing

Day Twelve

Breakfast

Eggs and Turkey

- 3 egg whites
- 2 oz. turkey
- ½ cup berries
- 1 cup cooked oatmeal

Snack

Protein shake or snack alternative

Lunch

Shrimp Salad

- 4 oz. cooked shrimp
- 3 cups lettuce
- ¼ cup cherry tomatoes
- ¼ cup slices cucumber
- 1 tsp low-fat dressing

Snack

Protein shake or snack alternative

Dinner

Pan-Sautéed Fish

- 4 oz. white fish
- 2 cups mixed green beans, broccoli, and asparagus
- ½ cup brown rice
- 1 tsp olive oil

Day Thirteen

Breakfast

Protein Pancakes

- ½ cup pancake mix mixed with ½ cup protein powder, 1 tbsp vegetable oil, 1 egg, and ¾ cup skim milk
- ½ cup sliced strawberries
- ½ cup low-fat cottage cheese

Use half the mix to make two pancakes for today; refrigerate remaining mix in airtight container.

Snack

Protein shake or snack alternative

Lunch

Seared Sea Scallops

- 5 large scallops
- garlic and bell peppers sautéed in 1 tsp olive oil
- ½ cup brown rice

Snack

Protein shake or snack alternative

Dinner

Asian Stir-Fry

- 4 oz. firm tofu, drained and cubed, sautéed with 2–3 cups mixed veggies in 1 tsp sesame oil
- mixed green salad with 1 tbsp vinaigrette

Day Fourteen

Breakfast

Power Up

- 3 egg whites
- ½ cup cottage cheese
- 6 almonds
- 1 cup high-fiber cereal
- ½ cup fresh berries

Snack

Protein shake or snack alternative

Lunch

Tuna Sandwich

- 4 oz. low-sodium, water-packed tuna
- 1 slice whole-wheat toast, such as Ezekiel
- 1 cup carrots and tomato
- 1 cup salad greens
- 1 tsp each olive oil and balsamic vinegar

Snack

Protein shake or snack alternative

Dinner

Grilled Salmon Salad

- 4 oz. grilled salmon
- 2 cups mixed lettuce
- 5 grilled asparagus spears
- ½ cup cherry tomatoes
- 1 tbsp low-fat dressing

Day Fifteen

Breakfast

Egg-White Wrap

- 1 whole-wheat wrap
- 3 scrambled egg whites
- ½ cup cottage cheese
- 1 oz. reduced-fat cheddar cheese

Snack

Protein shake or snack alternative

Lunch

Chopped Chef Salad

- 2 cups romaine lettuce
- ½ cup chopped cucumbers
- ¼ cup halved cherry tomatoes
- 2 hard-boiled eggs with one yolk removed, chopped
- 3 oz. chopped turkey
- 2 tbsp low-fat crumbled blue cheese
- 1 tbsp low-fat dressing

Snack

Protein shake or snack alternative

Dinner

Poached Halibut

- 4 oz. halibut fillet poached for approx. 10 min. in boiling water
- mixed, steamed vegetables such as baby carrots and cauliflower

Day Sixteen

Breakfast

Whole-Wheat French Toast

- 1 slice whole-wheat toast soaked in 1 beaten egg
- 1 cup low-fat milk cook as before and serve with
- 1 cup berries
- ½ cup cottage cheese

Snack

Protein shake or snack alternative

Lunch

Asian Chicken Salad

- 4 oz. grilled chicken
- sliced water chestnuts
- carrots, scallions, cucumbers
- 2 tsp sesame oil and brown rice vinegar
- lemon juice
- 12 peanuts

Snack

Protein shake or snack alternative

Dinner

Pork Tenderloin

- 4 oz. pork tenderloin roasted for 15 minutes at 350 degrees in paprika
- large mixed-green salad with cherry tomatoes and 1 tbsp low-fat vinaigrette

Day Seventeen

Breakfast

Eggs and Turkey

- 3 egg whites
- 2 oz. turkey
- ½ cup berries
- 1 cup cooked oatmeal

Snack

Protein shake or snack alternative

Lunch

Chicken Pita

- 1 small, whole-wheat pita pocket
- 2 tbsp hummus
- 1 cup shredded carrot and celery
- 4 oz. low-sodium chicken breast

Snack

Protein shake or snack alternative

Dinner

Pan-Sautéed Fish

- 4 oz. white fish
- 2 cups mixed green beans, broccoli, and asparagus, steamed or sautéed with the fish.
- ½ cup brown rice
- 1 tsp olive oil

Day Eighteen

Breakfast

Oatmeal with Apple, Nuts, and Cinnamon

- ½ cup oatmeal cooked with water and topped with 7 chopped walnuts, ½ cup chopped apple, and a dash of cinnamon
- 3 egg whites, scrambled

Snack

Protein shake or snack alternative

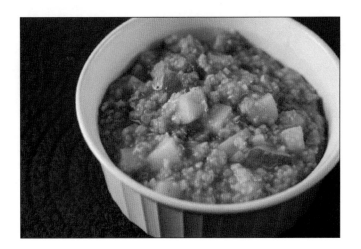

Lunch

Turkey Wrap

- 4 oz. turkey
- 1 whole-wheat tortilla
- 1 cup mixed greens
- ½ sliced avocado
- 1 tbsp balsamic vinaigrette

Snack

Protein shake or snack alternative

Dinner

Grilled Salmon Salad

- 4 oz. grilled salmon
- 2 cups romaine lettuce
- 1 oz. reduced-fat feta cheese
- ½ cup cherry tomatoes
- 1 tbsp low-fat dressing

Day Nineteen

Breakfast

Veggie Omelet

- 1 whole egg and 3 egg whites
- organic cooking spray
- 1 cup spinach, ½ chopped tomato, and 1 cup chopped mushrooms
- 1 slice whole-wheat toast, such as Ezekiel

Snack

Protein shake or snack alternative

Lunch

Tuna Sandwich

- 4 oz. low-sodium, water-packed tuna
- 1 slice whole-wheat toast, such as Ezekiel
- 1 cup carrots and tomato
- 1 cup salad greens
- 1 tsp each olive oil and balsamic vinegar

Snack

Protein shake or snack alternative

Dinner

Chicken Kebabs

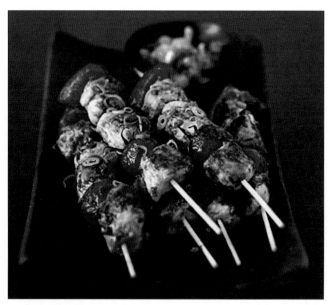

- 4 oz. chicken breast cut into cubes and skewered with mushrooms, green bell peppers, and cherry tomato
- large green salad with 1 tbsp low-fat dressing

Brush skewers with olive oil and grill over high heat 5–7 minutes.

Day Twenty

Breakfast

Eggs and Oats

- 3 egg whites
- ½ cup berries
- 1 cup cooked oatmeal
- 1 cup skim milk

Snack

Protein shake or snack alternative

Lunch

Turkey Burger

- 4 oz. ground lean turkey formed into a burger patty
- 1 whole-wheat burger bun
- ¼ sliced beefsteak tomato
- ½ sliced avocado
- small green salad

Snack

Protein shake or snack alternative

Dinner

Asian Stir-Fry

- 4 oz. firm tofu, drained and cubed, sautéed with 2–3 cups mixed veggies in 1 tsp sesame oil
- mixed green salad with 1 tbsp vinaigrette

Day Twenty-One

Breakfast

Waffle with Peanut Butter

- 1 whole-grain frozen waffle, such as Van's
- 2 tbsp natural peanut butter
- 1 cup skim milk
- 1 cup cut-up papaya

Snack

Protein shake or snack alternative

Lunch

Mediterranean Open-Faced Sandwich

- 2 tbsp hummus
- 2 tbsp guacamole
- 2 medium slices tomato
- lettuce to garnish
- 1 slice whole-grain bread, such as Ezekiel
- 3 slices low-sodium turkey breast

Snack

Protein shake or snack alternative

Dinner

Chicken with Greens

- 4 oz. broiled, skinless chicken breast
- 1 cup steamed broccoli
- 2 cups mixed greens with 1 tbsp low-fat balsamic dressing

Day Twenty-Two

Breakfast

Egg Muffin

- 1 whole-wheat English muffin
- 2 scrambled egg whites
- 2 large tomato slices
- ½ cup low-fat cottage cheese
- 6 walnuts

Snack

Protein shake or snack alternative

Lunch

Salad with Turkey

- 4 oz. cooked, chopped turkey breast
- 3 cups lettuce mix
- ¼ cup cherry tomatoes
- ¼ cup sliced cucumber
- ¼ cup chopped celery
- 1 tsp balsamic vinaigrette

Snack

Protein shake or snack alternative

Dinner

Shrimp Quinoa

- 4 oz. sautéed shrimp
- garlic and onion to taste
- 1 cup steamed asparagus
- ½ cup cooked quinoa
- sautéed sliced scallions and ½ sliced green bell pepper for garnish

Day Twenty-Three

Breakfast

Whole-Wheat French Toast

- 1 slice whole-wheat toast soaked in 1 beaten egg
- 1/2 cup low-fat milk
- 1 cup blueberries
- ½ cup cottage cheese

Snack

Protein shake or snack alternative

Lunch

Shrimp and Pasta

- ½ cup whole-wheat pasta, cooked
- 1 cup steamed asparagus
- 4 oz. boiled shrimp
- ½ cup marinara sauce *or* 2 tbsp pesto sauce
- pepper to taste

Snack

Protein shake or snack alternative

Dinner

Oriental Chicken Salad

- 4 oz. grilled chicken cooked in 1 tbsp coconut oil
- 12 peanuts combined with 1 cup water chestnuts, ¼ cup grated carrots, and sliced scallions served with
- 1 cup sliced cucumbers tossed in 1 tbsp low-fat dressing
- 2 cups salad greens

Day Twenty-Four

Breakfast

Waffle with Peanut Butter

- 1 whole-grain frozen waffle, such as Van's
- 2 tbsp natural peanut butter
- 1 small, low-fat cottage cheese cup
- 1/2 cup sliced banana

Snack

Protein shake or snack alternative

Lunch

Mediterranean Open-Faced Sandwich

- 1 slice whole-grain bread, such as Ezekiel
- 2 tbsp hummus
- 1/8 sliced avocado
- 2 medium slices tomato
- lettuce
- 3 slices low-sodium grilled turkey breast

Snack

Protein shake or snack alternative

Dinner

Chicken with Greens

- 4 oz. broiled, skinless chicken breast
- 2 cups mixed, steamed vegetables
- 2 cups mixed salad greens with 1 tbsp low-fat balsamic dressing

Day Twenty-Five

Breakfast

Yogurt with Granola

- ¼ cup low-sugar granola
- 1 cup plain Greek yogurt, such as Fage
- ½ cup berries
- 9 almonds, chopped

Snack

Protein shake or snack alternative

Lunch

Chopped Chef Salad

- 2 cups romaine lettuce
- ½ cup chopped cucumbers
- ¼ cup halved cherry tomatoes
- 2 hard-boiled eggs with one yolk removed, chopped
- 3 oz. chopped turkey
- 2 tbsp low-fat crumbled blue cheese
- 1 tbsp low-fat dressing

Snack

Protein shake or snack alternative

Dinner

Grilled Steak Fajitas

- 4 oz. lean beef tenderloin, cut into strips and sautéed
- red and green bell peppers, cut into strips and sautéed
- ½ onion, sliced and sautéed
- 1 cup mushrooms, sliced and sautéed
- 1 tbsp olive oil or spray for sautéing
- ½ cup brown rice or quinoa

Day Twenty-Six

Breakfast

Protein Pancakes

- ½ cup pancake mix mixed with ½ cup protein powder, 1 tbsp vegetable oil, 1 egg, and ¾ cup skim milk
- ½ cup sliced strawberries
- ½ cup low-fat cottage cheese

Use half the mix to make two pancakes for today; refrigerate remaining mix in airtight container.

Snack

Protein shake or snack alternative

Lunch

Chicken Pita

- 1 small, whole-wheat pita pocket
- 2 tbsp hummus
- 1 cup shredded carrot and celery
- 4 oz. low-sodium chicken breast, cut into strips
- lettuce

Snack

Protein shake or snack alternative

Dinner

Seared Sea Scallops

- 5–6 large scallops seared in organic cooking spray
- garlic, sliced onions, and bell peppers sautéed in 1 tsp olive oil
- ½ cup brown rice, pre cooked
- 1 handful sliced almonds to top it off

Day Twenty-Seven

Breakfast

Veggie Omelet

- 1 whole egg and ½ cup liquid egg whites
- organic cooking spray
- 1 cup spinach, ½ chopped tomato, and 1 cup chopped mushrooms
- seasoning
- 1 slice whole-wheat toast, such as Ezekiel

Snack

Protein shake or snack alternative

Lunch

Chicken Tortilla

- 1 whole-wheat tortilla
- 4 oz. grilled chicken
- chopped bell peppers, artichoke hearts, and tomatoes
- 1 tbsp low-fat dressing or fresh salsa to taste
- carrot and celery sticks on the side

Snack

Protein shake or snack alternative

Dinner

Asian Stir-Fry

- 4 oz. firm tofu, drained and cubed, sautéed with 2–3 cups mixed veggies in 1 tsp sesame oil
- small mixed-green salad with 1 tbsp vinaigrette

Day Twenty-Eight

Breakfast

Egg Muffin

- 1 whole-wheat English muffin
- 2 scrambled egg whites
- 2 large tomato slices
- ½ cup low-fat cottage cheese
- 6 walnuts

Snack

Protein shake or snack alternative

Lunch

Salad with Turkey

- 4 oz. cooked turkey
- 3 cups mixed lettuce
- ¼ cup cherry tomatoes
- ¼ cup sliced cucumber
- balsamic vinegar and seasonings to taste

Snack

Protein shake or snack alternative

Dinner

Shrimp with Quinoa

- 4 oz. sautéed shrimp
- garlic and onion to taste
- 1 cup steamed broccoli
- ½ cup cooked quinoa
- sautéed scallions and green bell peppers for garnish

You Made It—Now Reward Yourself!

I am so happy for you! Now you've learned what it takes to eat healthy for the rest of your life. You should be feeling better, sleeping better, having more energy throughout your day, and looking leaner and fitter than just a few short weeks ago. *Reward yourself by getting a facial or a massage, buying a new outfit, or enjoying an activity you have been putting off.* Do not reward yourself with food. You've learned that food can be a great source of comfort and sustenance, but you do not want to associate rewards with food.

This advice is also true when it comes to your children. Avoid teaching your children that food is something other than fuel for your body. This way you will not fall into the trap of a downward spiral where you start eating foods that damage your health and your waistline. Your taste buds have now been "reset" to appreciate cleaner, healthier foods. Stick to your healthy eating pattern, and choose to reward yourself with meaningful or joyful experiences instead of food, sweets, or alcohol.

The Maintenance Phase

Congratulations! You made it to your goal weight. *This is a huge accomplishment*, and I'm sure that you are feeling better than ever. The important thing is for you to keep your metabolism revved up while *slowly* adding some more calories back into your diet. It is important that you add calories slowly and that you keep monitoring your weight weekly. This way, you will be able to assess how you are doing and to address any weight fluctuations as soon as possible.

Since the meal plan you have been on is very sound nutritionally, and also very nutrient dense, I would recommend that it become your *way of life. The way to maintain your new weight is to follow the meal plan and also allow yourself an occasional "cheat" meal, while knowing how to make up for it.* The best way to do this is to add a high-carb, higher-calorie day about once a week. This will keep your leptin levels high, thereby preventing lower metabolic rate and increased hunger.

By now you know what makes up a healthy meal, and you also know that you need to eat every three hours. That will not change. If you allow yourself a "cheat meal," the best way to compensate for this is to increase your activity and cut back on your calories slightly the very next day. Occasional "cheat meals" are actually good for you, at this point, as they keep your body "guessing," preventing it from going into a plateau. The important thing is that after you have your "cheat meal," you get right back on the meal plan.

Chapter 18: The "Diet Diva" 1,200-Calorie, Seven-Day Metabolism-Igniter Meal Plan

This is the fat-melting plan you should be on when you are serious about jump-starting your fat loss and gaining sleek, sexy muscle in no time. *Remember, 1,200 calories is at the lower range of what is considered safe to consume before you start negatively affecting your metabolism, so be sure to eat all your meals as suggested.*

The meals on this plan are all composed of approximately 30 percent complex carbohydrates consumed early in the day, 40 percent protein, and 30 percent "healthy" fats.

On this meal plan, you should make sure to take a daily multivitamin; as always, *stay clear of sugar, sweets, and alcohol*; and restrict your sodium intake as well as drinking at least eight to ten glasses of water per day. Please consult with a physician before starting any diet or exercise program.

You need to *stay consistent*. Stick to the plan. *There is not a lot of variety, but you will boost your metabolic rate significantly.* Stick to the timing as well. *You* must *eat every three hours, starting with breakfast within half an hour of waking up to get your metabolism going.*

Eat all your meals. Your meals are fueling your revved-up metabolism. To keep the fire burning, you have to fuel it. **Do not skip meals!** *This is essential!*

Stick to the right foods. On this meal plan I do not recommend cruciferous veggies, and your protein sources should be lean and clean.

Make sure you *drink as much water as possible*. I suggest at least *one hundred ounces per day*. That is roughly five to six medium-sized water bottles per day. This will improve your metabolic rate as well. You may become very familiar with the bathroom, but that's a great sign that your metabolism is revving up and you are shedding fat!

Exercise. It is *imperative* that you increase your activity level to burn your stored energy (fat) to lose the maximum amount of fat. Exercise for at least forty-five minutes five times per week. Do something even if you don't have forty-five minutes. In the exercise section of this book, I will outline workouts that have proven highly effective in sculpting every single muscle group in your body and at the same time burn the maximum amount of fat. If you have only twenty minutes, then do what you can in that time. *Just get it done.*

The most difficult day is the first one. Once you get into the habit of working out, you will actually look forward to it, and love and embrace the way it makes you feel. Believe me, I have been there: exhausted from my responsibilities, with no desire to get into my gym clothes and do a workout. But you know what? Within just a few minutes of getting started, I already feel better. The endorphins that are released in the body in response to physical activity are so comforting. You feel more energized yet at the same time more relaxed.

I recommend that you do a high-intensity training program such as the JNL Fusion Program, which is the *best* way to *melt fat while getting lean muscle tone*. Alternatively you may walk at a brisk pace, bike, jog, swim, or use cardio equipment. When you want maximum results in minimum time, you should try HIIT, which is discussed later in this book. You should be able to keep a slightly breathless conversation while exercising or when doing your "recovery" periods in HIIT. This ensures that you are not working too hard and depriving your body of oxygen, thereby burning your muscle instead of your fat stores.

While I suggest a *protein shake or snack alternative* made with a high-quality, no -sugar protein powder such as the BodyFX products and water for your midmorning and/or midafternoon snack, you can also eat other snacks, such as the following "Diet Diva Approved" snacks:

Alternative Snacks

- celery or carrot sticks with 2 tablespoons peanut or almond butter
- 1 high-quality, low-sugar protein bar such as "NuGo Slim" or "Think Thin"
- 1 small handful of high-quality, unsalted, natural nuts, such as almonds, walnuts, or cashews
- 1 low-fat cheese stick with 5–7 whole-wheat, low-sodium crackers
- 1–2 hard-boiled eggs, yolks removed, and 1 cup of raw veggies
- 5-7 crackers with 2 tablespoons hummus or natural nut butter
- 2 low-sodium rice cakes with 1 tablespoon almond or peanut butter or 1 cup low-fat organic cottage cheese
- ½ cup nonfat Greek yogurt with 3 tablespoons wheat germ or ½ cup low-sugar, high-protein cereal

The Meal Plan
(supports a woman weighing 125 pounds or more)

Day One
Breakfast

- 1 egg, 4 egg whites, or ½ cup liquid egg whites
- ½ cup instant oatmeal mixed with water
- ¼ sliced banana
- black coffee or green tea

233 calories, 9 g fat, 23 g protein, 30 g carbohydrates, 287 mg sodium

Snack

Protein shake or snack alternative

150 calories, 2 g fat, 23 g protein, 3 g carbohydrates, 150 mg sodium

Lunch

- 4 oz. skinless chicken breast or fish, grilled or steamed
- ½ cup brown rice
- 1 cup asparagus
- 2 cups green salad
- 1 tbsp low-calorie dressing or balsamic vinegar with 1 tsp olive oil

333 calories, 5 g fat, 30 g protein, 31 g carbohydrates, 229 mg sodium

Snack

Protein shake or snack alternative

150 calories, 2 g fat, 23 g protein, 3 g carbohydrates, 150 mg sodium

Dinner

- 4 oz. grilled, skinless chicken or turkey
- 1 cup zucchini
- 1 cup asparagus
- 3 cups mixed salad greens

260 calories, 2 g fat, 36 g protein, 25 g carbohydrates, 120 mg sodium

Daily: 1,246 calories, 20–24 g fat, 135 g protein, 92 g carbohydrates, 1,086 mg sodium

Day Two

Breakfast

- 1 cup liquid egg whites
- 1 cup spinach
- ½ toasted whole-grain English muffin
- black coffee or green tea

267 calories, 3 g fat, 33 g protein, 30 g carbs, 287 sodium

Snack

Protein shake or snack alternative

150 calories, 2 g fat, 23 g protein, 3 g carbohydrates, 150 mg sodium

Lunch

- 4 oz. water-packed tuna, rinsed and drained
- ½ whole-grain pita pocket
- 1 cup sliced red pepper and shredded carrot
- 2 cups green salad
- 1 tbsp low-calorie dressing

314 calories, 5 g fat, 43 g protein, 26 g carbohydrates, 229 mg sodium

Snack

Protein shake or snack alternative

150 calories, 2 g fat, 23 g protein, 3 g carbohydrates, 150 mg sodium

Dinner

- 5 oz. tilapia, oven baked or sautéed in 1 tsp olive oil
- 1 cup sautéed sliced vegetables
- 2 tbsp tomato sauce
- 2 cups green salad

292 calories, 4 g fat, 37 g protein, 30 g carbohydrates, 120 mg sodium

Daily: 1,212 calories, 21 g fat, 135 g protein, 99 g carbohydrates, 1,086 mg sodium

Day Three

Breakfast

- 1 slice whole-wheat toast
- 3 slices low-sodium turkey breast
- 2 slices beefsteak tomato
- black coffee or green tea

349 calories, 4 g fat, 39 g protein, 39 g carbohydrates, 287 mg sodium

Snack

Protein shake or snack alternative

150 calories, 2 g fat, 23 g protein, 3 g carbohydrates, 150 mg sodium

Lunch

- 4 oz. grilled chicken
- ½ cup brown rice
- 1 chopped tomato
- 2 cups shredded lettuce
- 1 tbsp low-calorie dressing
- 1 tbsp salsa

262 calories, 4 g fat, 29 g protein, 27.6 g carbohydrates, 229 mg sodium

Snack

Protein shake or snack alternative

150 calories, 2 g fat, 23 g protein, 3 g carbohydrates, 150 mg sodium

Dinner

- 4 oz. grilled or baked skinless turkey
- 3 cups salad greens
- 1 tbsp low-calorie salad dressing

260 calories, 2 g fat, 26 g protein, 25 g carbohydrates, 120 mg sodium

Daily: 1,171 calories, 14 g fat, 115 g protein, 88 g carbohydrates, 936 mg sodium

Day Four

Breakfast

- 1 egg, 3 egg whites, or ½ cup liquid egg whites
- ½ cup instant oatmeal mixed with water
- black coffee or green tea

213 calories, 9 g fat, 17 g protein, 33 g carbohydrates, 287 mg sodium

Snack

Protein shake or snack alternative

150 calories, 2 g fat, 23 g protein, 3 g carbohydrates, 150 mg sodium

Lunch

- 4 oz. grilled chicken
- ½ cup brown rice
- 1 chopped tomato
- 2 cups shredded lettuce
- 1 tbsp low-calorie dressing
- 1 tbsp salsa

270 calories, 3 g fat, 30 g protein, 33 g carbohydrates, 229 mg sodium

Snack

Protein shake or snack alternative

150 calories, 2 g fat, 23 g protein, 3 g carbohydrates, 150 mg sodium

Dinner

- 5 oz. tilapia, oven baked or sautéed in olive oil spray
- 1 cup sautéed sliced vegetables
- 2 tbsp low-sugar tomato sauce
- 2 cups green salad

355 calories, 4 g fat, 39 g protein, 25 g carbohydrates, 120 mg sodium

Daily: 1,149 calories, 22.8 g fat, 108 g protein, 92 g carbohydrates, 936 mg sodium

Day Five

Breakfast

- ½ cup egg whites
- ½ cup spinach
- ½ toasted whole grain English muffin
- black coffee or green tea

267 calories, 2 g fat, 33 g protein, 30 g carbohydrates, 287 mg sodium

Snack:

Protein shake or snack alternative

150 calories, 2 g fat, 23 g protein, 3 g carbohydrates, 150 mg sodium

Lunch

4 oz. sliced, grilled turkey breast

½ whole-grain pita pocket

2 slices tomato

2 cups green salad

1 tbsp low-calorie dressing

314 calories, 5 g fat, 43 g protein, 26 g carbohydrates, 229 mg sodium

Snack

Protein shake or snack alternative

150 calories, 2 g fat, 23 g protein, 3 g carbohydrates, 150 mg sodium

Dinner

- 5 oz. grilled chicken
- 1 cup zucchini
- 1 cup asparagus
- 3 cups mixed salad greens

292 calories, 4 g fat, 36 g protein, 25 g carbohydrates, 120 mg sodium

Daily: 1,149 calories, 22.8 g fat, 108 g protein, 92 g carbohydrates, 936 mg sodium

Day Six

Breakfast

- 1 whole-grain frozen waffle
- 1 tbsp natural peanut butter
- 1 cup skim milk
- 1 cup cut-up papaya

315 calories, 9.9 g fat, 15 g protein, 45 g carbs, 120 mg sodium

Snack

Protein shake or snack alternative

150 calories, 2 g fat, 23 g protein, 3 g carbohydrates, 150 mg sodium

Lunch

- 4 oz. grilled chicken breast
- ½ cup quinoa
- 1 chopped tomato
- 2 cups shredded lettuce
- 1 tbsp low-calorie dressing
- 1 tbsp salsa

266 calories, 5 g fat, 30 g protein, 31 g carbs, 429 mg sodium

Snack

Protein shake or snack alternative

150 calories, 2 g fat, 23 g protein, 3 g carbohydrates, 150 mg sodium

Dinner

- 4 oz. tilapia, oven baked or sautéed in olive oil
- 1 cup sautéed sliced vegetables
- 2 tbsp low-sugar tomato sauce
- 2 cups green salad

260 calories, 2 g fat, 36 g protein, 25 g carbohydrates, 120 mg sodium

Daily: 1,149 calories, 28.2 g fat, 103 g protein, 115 g carbohydrates, 969 mg sodium

Day Seven

Breakfast

- 1 cup plain Greek yogurt
- ½ cup low-sugar, high-protein granola
- ½ cup egg whites
- coffee or green tea

263 calories, 2 g fat, 36 g protein, 20 g carbohydrates, 320 mg sodium

Snack

Protein shake or snack alternative

150 calories, 2 g fat, 23 g protein, 3 g carbohydrates, 150 mg sodium

Lunch

- 1.5 cups low-sodium tomato soup
- 1 slice whole-wheat toast
- 3 oz. sliced low-fat cheese
- 2 large slices tomato
- lettuce

341 calories, 6 g fat, 31 g protein, 40 g carbohydrates, 150 mg sodium

Snack

Protein shake or snack alternative

150 calories, 2 g fat, 23 g protein, 3 g carbohydrates, 150 mg sodium

Dinner

- 4 oz. lean beef cut into strips
- 2 cups sautéed sliced mixed vegetables
- ½ cup onion
- 1 tbsp olive oil
- ½ cup brown rice

480 calories, 5 g fat, 34 g protein, 28 g carbohydrates, 200 mg sodium

Daily: 1,240 calories, 20.2 g fat, 128 g protein, 96 g carbohydrates, 1,270 mg sodium

This meal plan can be repeated for as long as it takes you to get to your goal weight. Once you reach your goal weight, it is very important to *slowly increase the amount of food that you consume daily.* You must ease yourself into a "maintenance" phase of at least a few weeks to stabilize your weight. When you see that you have kept your goal weight for at least a month, you may add weekly cheat meals and occasional treats.

Part IV

Exercise

Even though diet makes up 80 percent of how we look and feel, we can't forget the importance of exercise. As you already know, I am a certified master trainer, and I spend most of my time in my gym, either training clients or working out myself. I love to work out! Really, I do. There is no better feeling than how you feel after a great workout. Your body is made to move and to go through pushing and pulling, jumping, skipping, and working up a good sweat.

For optimal health, I say you need to *aim for a good sweat five to six days a week.* Just as with food and nutrition, I have tried countless workout methods and modalities over the last forty or so years, on myself as well as on others, and I have come to some important conclusions.

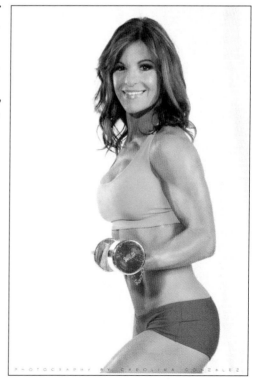

Weight Training

As you have learned, it is essential for you to build lean mass in order to increase your metabolic rate. The best and quickest way to build lean mass is by *weight or resistance training.* Many women are afraid of weight training, as they fear that they will become large or "bulky." Some of my own clients express this fear. It is simply impossible for a woman to grow large muscle mass naturally. As we previously discussed, women have high levels of estrogen. Our bodies are naturally primed for reproduction, and that is why we carry more body fat and generally appear "softer" than men. In contrast, men produce more of the hormone *testosterone*, which is essential for muscle building. Due to this naturally occurring testosterone, it is much easier for men to get "big" and lean.

You will alternate between upper-body and lower-body workouts to give your muscles a chance to recover for at least twenty-four hours before that same muscle is worked again. On some days you may choose a full-body workout, which is another way to slightly increase your caloric burn over just training one body part.

Interval Training

Studies show that *interval training burns more fat than slow or steady-state cardio*. In fact, not only do you torch more *fat* during your high-intensity training (HIIT) workout, but *your metabolism also stays elevated for as much as sixteen to eighteen hours afterward*.

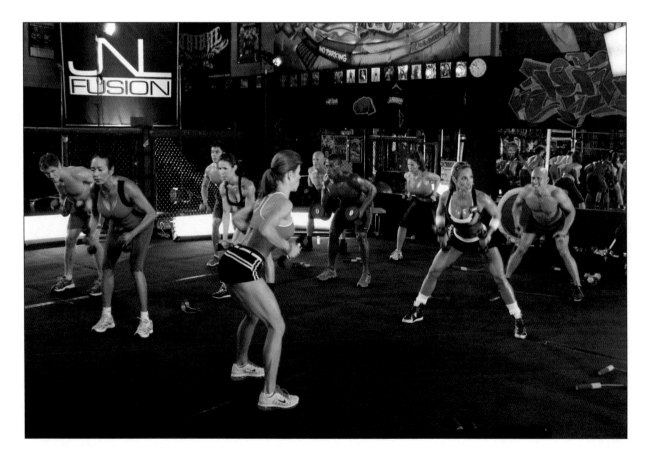

One way to incorporate interval training is to *combine* your weight training with cardio bursts in between sets. I have had the privilege of working alongside Jennifer Nicole Lee for years. As you may know, she pioneered the JNL Fusion workout method and DVD set. Her revolutionary workout method combines weight training and cardio and is highly effective. Through this method, you "super spike" your metabolism and build lean, sexy muscle at the same time, in quick, fun workouts. You will not believe your eyes when you see the results that you will achieve. This program is wonderful, because it can be done anywhere by anyone at anytime! The Fusion method can be done at any fitness level from the novice exerciser to the advanced athlete, with stunning results. Since you only need a few dumbbells or resistance bands, you can do it anywhere.

Before you start any workout program, it is important that you get clearance from your doctor or licensed health-care practitioner. You should start each workout with a warm-up and stretching. This will get the blood flowing to your muscles, and you will be ready for the more challenging part of the workout, without the risk of injury or strain.

As you do the workouts, perform at least twelve to fifteen reps of each exercise for three sets. If you are looking to really build mass, lower your rep range to no more than ten reps and lift as heavy as possible. To tone up and slim down, go for a higher rep range with a weight that you can handle. Personally, I do up to twenty repetitions per set. The last three reps should become fairly difficult to finish. If they are too easy, you need to add more weight so that you keep challenging your muscle tissue.

After each set, you will do a "cardio burst" for thirty seconds. I use a Gymboss timer to count down my cardio interval. You can order your own Gymboss timer at www.unnigreene.com.

Whenever you are weight training, be mindful of your posture. Always think of standing erect with knees slightly bent, abs and core engaged, and your shoulder blades retracted so that your chest is open. I want you to use full range of motion in each exercise, meaning that you should fully extend your arms on the lengthening or eccentric part of the exercise, and always squeeze on the concentric part or "finish." Pause as you contract your muscle fully for a count of two, and then slowly bring the weight back to starting position.

Remember, always start every workout with a five-minute warm-up and stretching sessions. Gather your equipment, a towel, and some water to stay hydrated. Then do three to four sets of at least twelve but no more than twenty reps of everything. The last three reps should be challenging. Pick a weight that's heavy enough!

Chapter 19: Total Body Workout

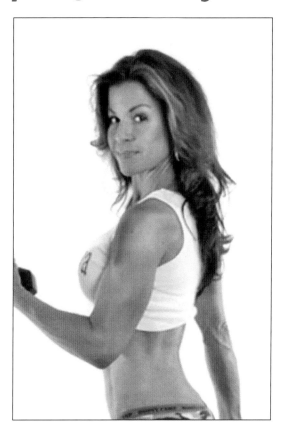

Always start every workout with a five-minute warm-up and stretching sessions. Gather your equipment, a towel, and some water to stay hydrated. Then do three to four sets of at least twelve but no more than twenty reps of everything. The last three reps should be challenging. Pick a weight that's heavy enough!

In all the exercises, make sure that you bend your knees and engage your core by keeping your abdominals tight. Tuck your butt in and down. Do each rep slowly, and concentrate on putting your mind in the muscle that you are working.

Squats

Stand erect with your feet slightly wider than shoulder width apart. Toes should be pointing slightly out. Keep your head up, back arched, and chest up. Grab your dumbbells and, with your body weight on your heels, slowly lower yourself by bending your knees and pushing your glutes back. Lower until you are parallel with the floor and your knees are at a ninety-degree angle. Pause and push back up to standing. As you get to the top of the move, squeeze your glutes hard. Repeat for reps.

Research shows that muscles engage 30 percent more when you think about the muscle you are working as opposed to letting your mind wander, so put your mind in your muscle!

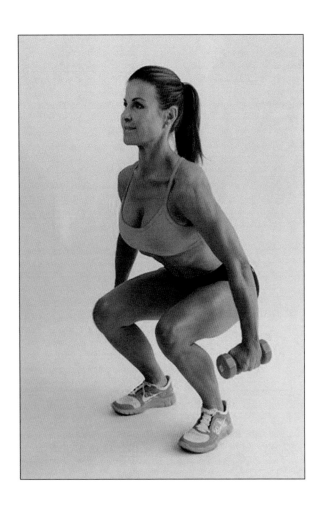
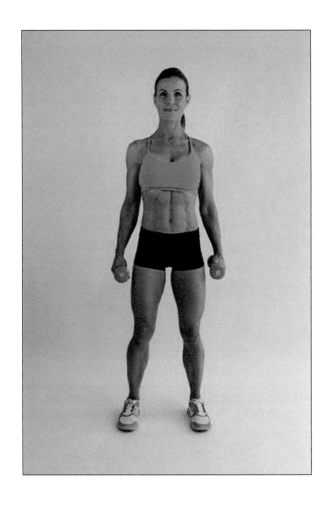

Jumping Jacks

The old-school cardio igniter is back! Set your Gymboss or count out loud to thirty. Go the full range of motion, making sure that your fingertips touch as you swing your arms overhead, and that you jump out as wide as possible while remaining comfortable.

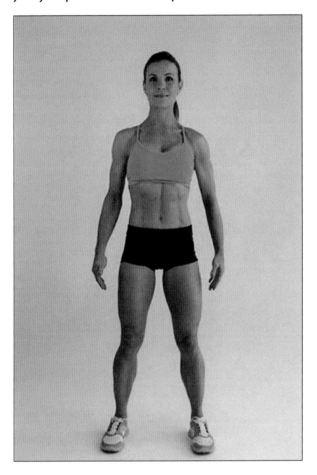 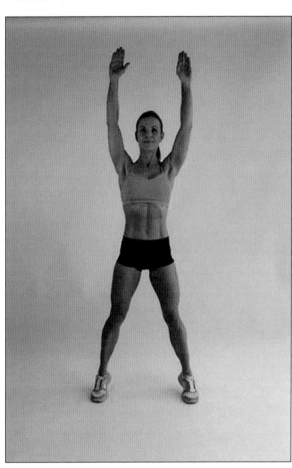

Repeat squats and jumping jacks for a total of three times each.

Shoulder Press

Grab your dumbbells. Stand with feet shoulder width apart, knees slightly bent. Hold the dumbbells just above your shoulders, palms facing each other. Engage your core and squeeze your glutes. Press the weights up until your arms are straight. Pause, then slowly return to starting position. Repeat for reps.

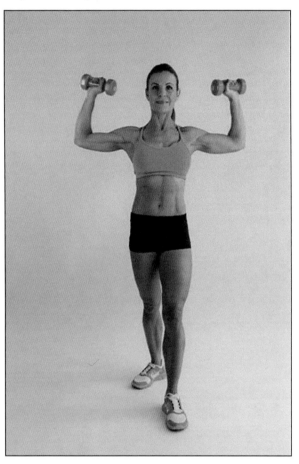 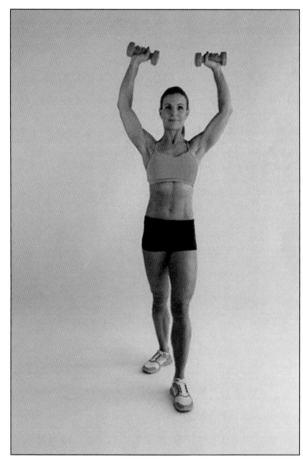

High Knees

Stand erect with your feet wider than shoulder width apart. Toes should be pointing straight forward. Go into a fast jog, bringing your knees up as high as possible while simultaneously pumping your arms. Go for thirty seconds. Repeat for a total of three times each.

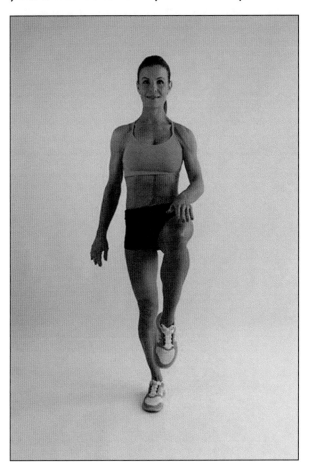 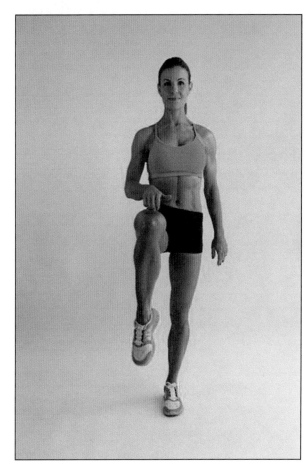

Step Out, Alternating Lunges

Stand erect with your feet wider than shoulder width apart. Toes should be pointing straight forward. Keep your head up, back arched, and chest up. Grab your dumbbells and with your body weight on your heels step out with one foot forward into a lunge. Lower yourself until your front knee forms a ninety-degree angle and your back knee is only slightly off the ground. Push back up with your front leg, focusing on pushing through the heel, and return to standing. Repeat with the other leg. Continue until you have completed twenty reps on each leg.

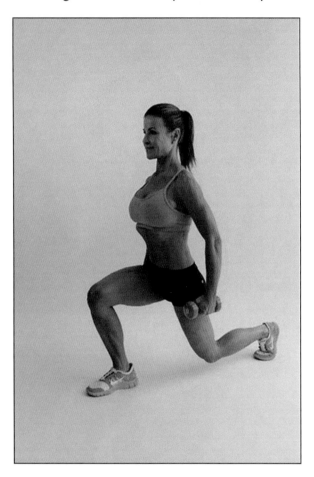
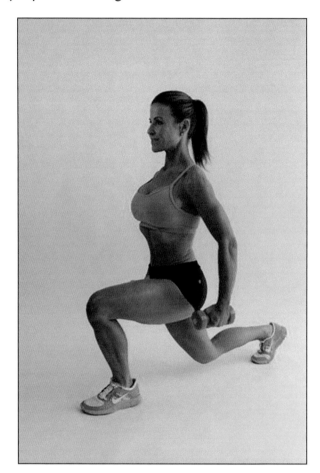

Half Burpees

Squat down to a deep squat, with knees touching your elbows. Touch the ground with your hands firmly planted, and explode, bringing your legs out directly behind you as far as you can, forming a plank. Bring legs back to starting position. Repeat for thirty seconds.

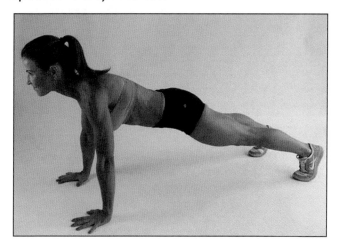

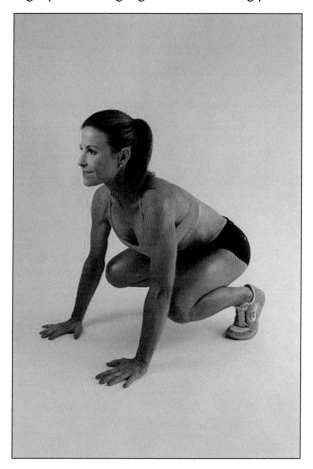

Repeat for a total of three times each.

Shoulder Side Raises

Stand erect with your feet shoulder width apart. Toes should be pointing straight forward. Keep your head up, back arched, and chest up. Grasp dumbbells in front of thighs, palms facing each other and elbows slightly bent. Bend over slightly with hips and knees bent slightly. Engage your core and glutes. Raise upper arms to sides until elbows are shoulder height. Maintain elbows' height above or equal to wrists. Briefly pause on top. Lower and repeat for reps.

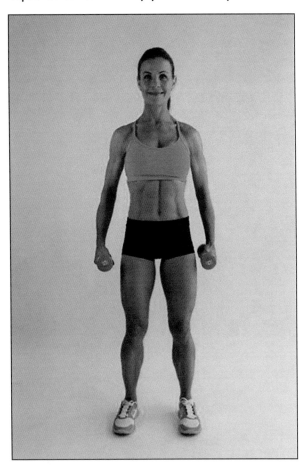
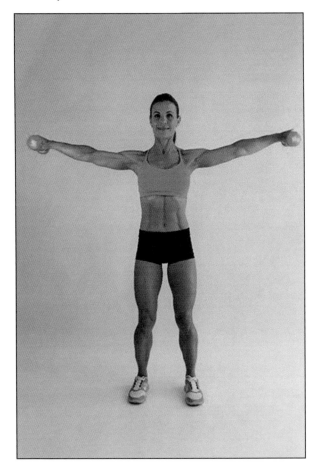

Scissors

Stand with feet together. Put one leg in front of the other, with knees slightly bent. One arm starts over your head, and the other arm is down, elbows slightly bent. Switch arms from above to below, alternating your legs at the same time. You need to exert force from your legs as you hop up and make the switch in midair. Land gently with soft knees. Continue for thirty seconds.

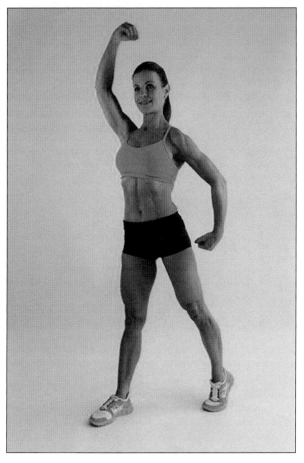 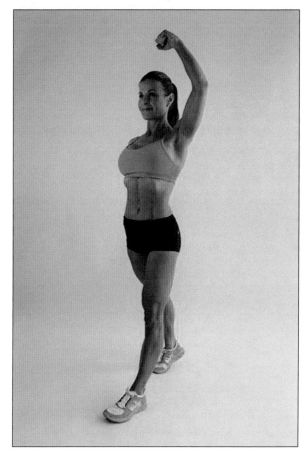

Repeat for a total of three times each.

Upright Rows

Stand erect with your feet shoulder width apart. Toes should be pointing straight forward. Keep your head up, back arched, and chest up. Grasp dumbbells in front of thighs, palms facing each other and elbows slightly bent. Pull the dumbbell up toward your collarbone, keeping it close to your body as you lift. Lead with your elbows so that at the top of the move, the elbows are slightly higher than your wrist. Pause briefly, and then return to starting position. Repeat for reps.

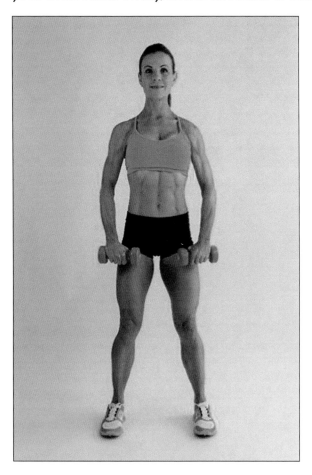
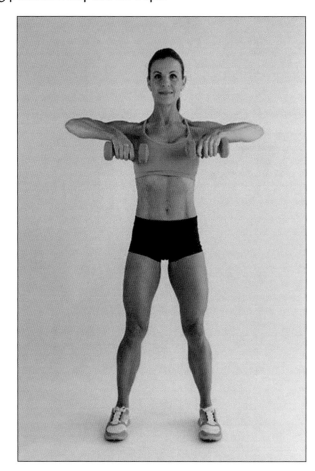

Jump Rope

This is a great cardio burst that you can do with or even without a jump rope. Skip for thirty seconds as you keep your elbows close to your waist, while rotating your arms. Jump about one-quarter to one-half inch off the ground, no more, and land softly on the balls of your feet.

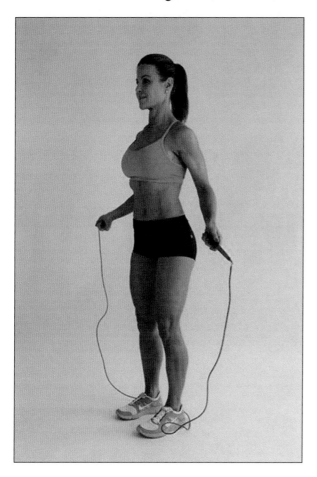

Jumping rope engages every muscle and helps develop agility, quickness, balance, speed, and conditioning. Jumping also improves bone density!

Ab Crunches

Lie on the floor on a mat or towel. Knees are bent, and lower back is pressed into the floor. Place your hands gently behind your neck, elbows pointing up and out. As you engage your abdominals, slowly raise your upper body off the floor while you exhale. Keep your neck flat, and don't pull your head forward. Your shoulder blades should come completely off the floor. When you reach the top, exhale and contract your abdominals. Hold briefly, then lower and repeat.

Rest for thirty seconds in between sets, and perform three sets of thirty crunches.

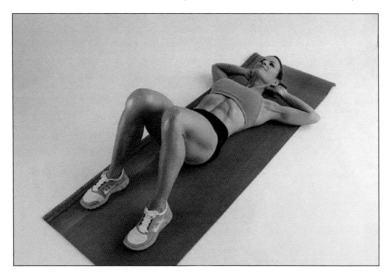

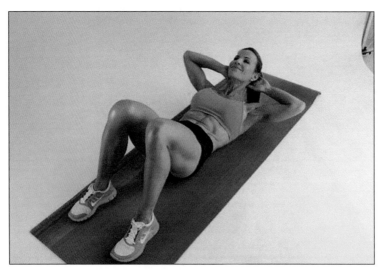

Russian Twists

Sit on the floor with your knees bent and your back flat. Hold your arms straight out, palms facing each other. Your torso should be forty-five degrees off the floor, and your feet should be slightly off the floor. As you balance on your glutes, slowly rotate to the right and try to touch the floor with your hands. Pause, and then reverse the movement, rotating to the left as far as you can. Repeat for thirty reps and three sets with no more than thirty seconds of rest between sets.

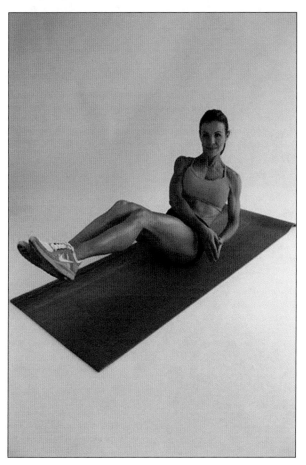
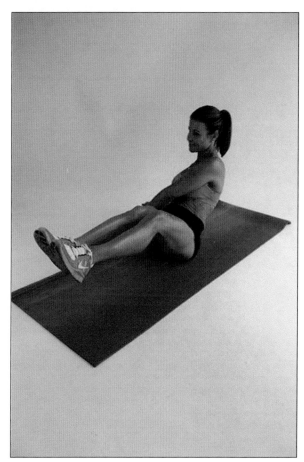

Raised-Leg Crunch

Lie on your back with your legs straight up and hips at ninety-degree angle. Place your arms at your sides, and slowly push your hips and glutes off the ground by contracting your lower abdominals. Keep your feet flexed and your legs straight. Do not swing your legs or use momentum. Repeat for twenty reps. Rest thirty seconds between sets and do three sets.

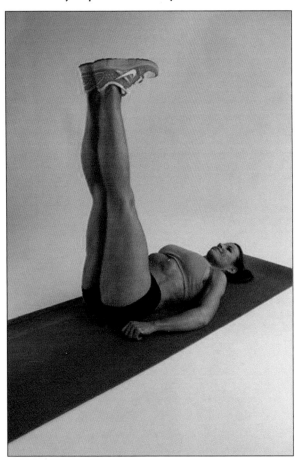 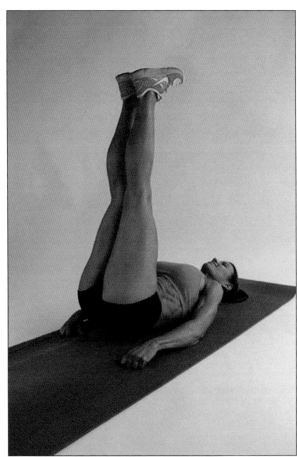

Cool Down and Stretch Out

Every workout session should be finished with a *cool down and stretching period of about three to five minutes.* It is very important to gradually bring your heart rate back down to normal and to stretch out the muscles you just worked so hard. Stretching prevents injury, speeds healing, and increases flexibility and overall joint mobility. As you do your stretches, make sure to challenge yourself to the point of slight discomfort, but never pain!

Always consume a high-quality hydrolyzed protein powder or other protein source within thirty minutes of finishing your workout, as this is the optimal time frame for refueling your muscles to repair and rebuild them.

Chapter 20: Upper Body Bicep, Triceps, and Glutes Workout

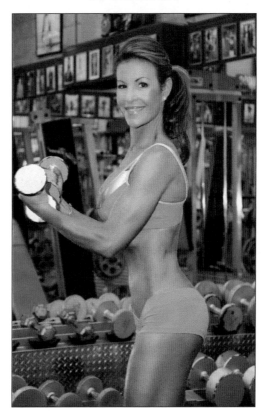

Always start every workout with a five-minute warm-up and stretching session. Gather your equipment, a towel, and some water to stay hydrated.

Perform three to four sets of at least twelve but no more than twenty reps of everything. The last three reps should be challenging. Pick a weight that's heavy enough to challenge you!

Bicep Curls

Stand erect with your feet shoulder width apart. Toes should be pointing straight forward and knees should be slightly bent. Keep your head up, back slightly arched, and chest elevated. Grasp dumbbells and extend arms fully in front of thighs, palms facing forward. Without moving your upper arms or your hips, slowly curl the weights up toward your shoulders. Pause at the top and squeeze your biceps, then slowly lower to starting position by completely straightening your arms. Repeat for reps.

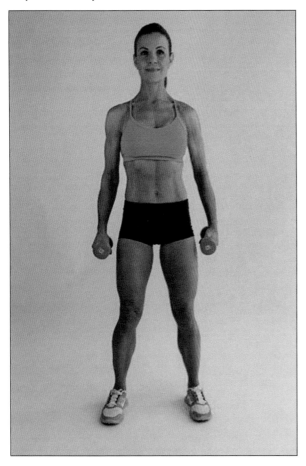 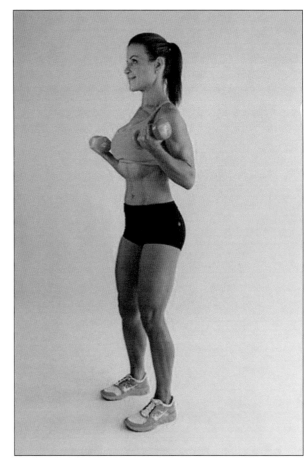

Jumping Jacks

Stand with your arms at your sides. Be sure your feet are straight and close together. Bend your knees slightly. Jump up while spreading your arms and legs at the same time. Lift your arms to your ears, and open your feet to a little wider than shoulder width. This should all be done in a fast, fluid movement. Touch your hands above your head. As you return from jumping up, bring your arms back down to your sides and at the same time bring your feet back together. Repeat for thirty seconds.

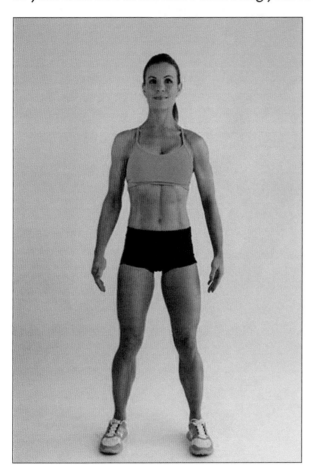 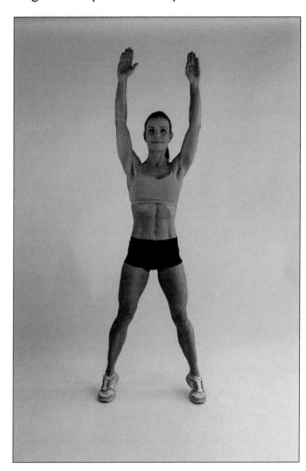

Hammer Curls

Stand erect with your feet shoulder width apart. Toes should be pointing straight forward and knees slightly bent. Keep your head up, back slightly arched, and chest elevated. Relax your arms down, with dumbbells in hands, palms facing in. Bring the top of each dumbbell up toward your shoulder, contracting hard at the top and slowly returning to start. Repeat for reps.

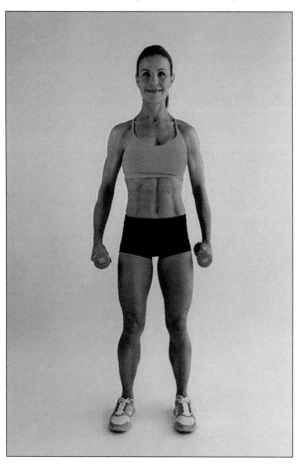
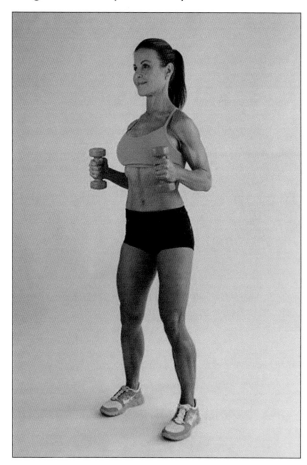

Squat Jumps

Stand with feet shoulder width apart, knees bent at ninety degrees. Explode up, pushing through your heels as you switch legs in midair. Land softly and repeat for thirty seconds.

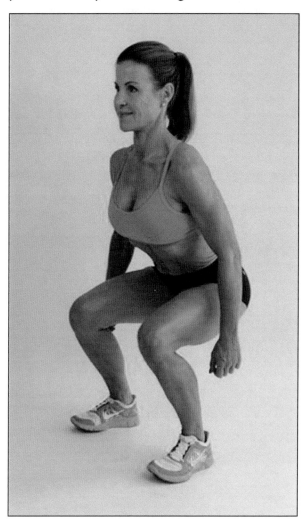
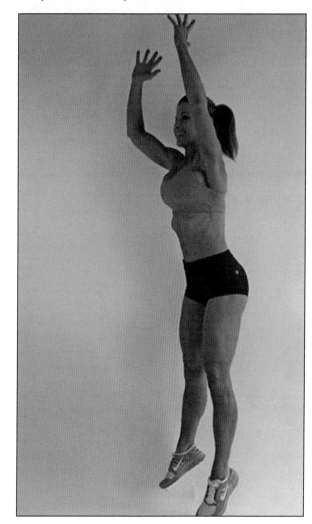

Bicep Curls with Hands Turned Out

Stand erect with your feet shoulder width apart. Toes should be pointing straight forward and knees slightly bent. Keep your head up, back slightly arched, and chest elevated. Relax your arms down; with dumbbells in hands, bend your elbows with palms facing up and out. Bring the top of each dumbbell up toward your shoulder, contracting hard at the top and slowly returning to start. Repeat for reps.

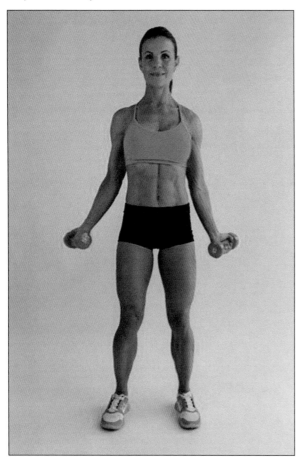
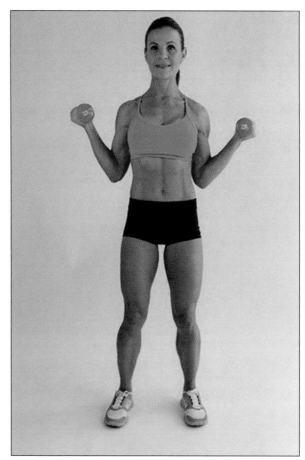

Triceps Overhead Press

Stand erect with your feet shoulder width apart. Toes should be pointing straight forward and knees should be slightly bent. Keep your head up, back slightly arched, and chest elevated. Place dumbbells in your hands and extend arms overhead. Raise arms, and then bend your elbows and put them very close to your ears, with hands behind your head. Slowly contract your triceps to bring your arms and hands directly over your head. Squeeze and slowly return to staring position. Repeat for reps.

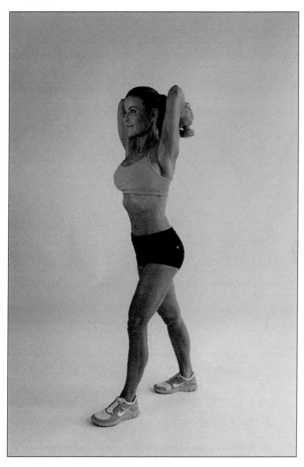
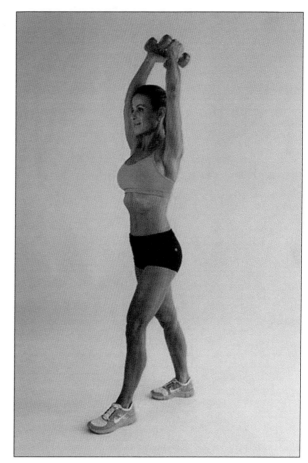

Mountain Climbers

Get into a plank position with legs fully extended behind you. Contract your abs, keeping your neck neutral and aligned with your upper body, and place the weight onto your arms. Quickly bring one knee at a time in toward your torso, while contracting your abs and alternating your legs. Continue for thirty seconds.

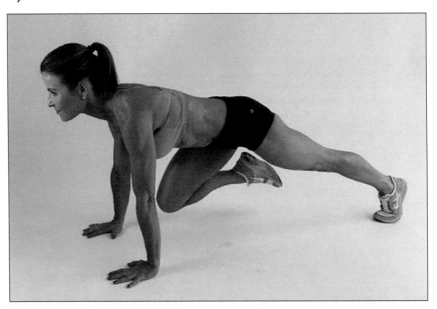

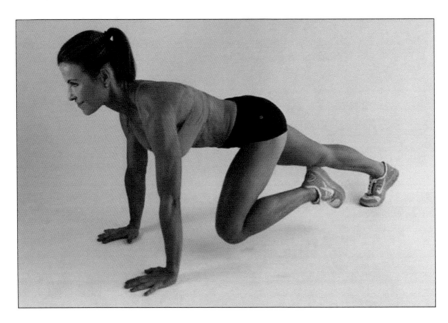

Triceps Kickbacks

Stand bent over at the waist with your feet shoulder width apart. Toes should be pointing straight forward and knees should be bent. Keep your head neutral, back slightly arched, and chest slightly elevated. Place dumbbells in your hands, and hold your upper arms parallel to your torso. Bend elbows at ninety degrees with hands by your thighs. Slowly push arms straight back and up toward the ceiling until entire arm is completely parallel to the floor. Squeeze the triceps hard and return slowly to start. Repeat for reps.

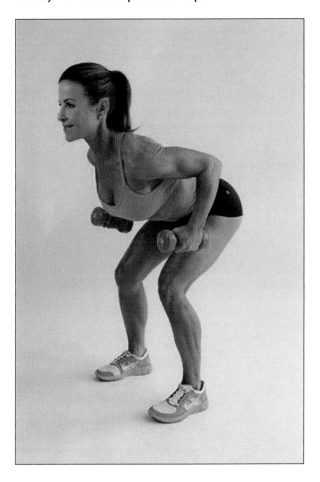 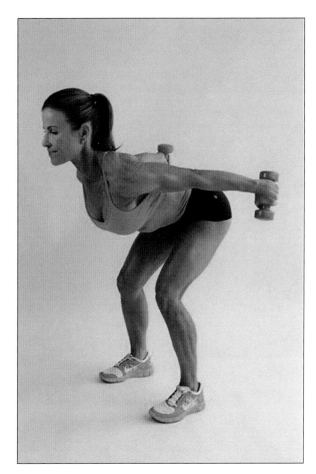

Jump Rope

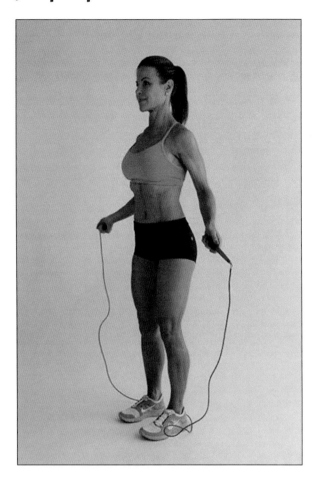

When you are working out, remember that quality is more important than quantity. That means that you should always strive to perfect your form, do each rep slowly, and concentrate on squeezing the muscle you are working.

Triceps Dips on Bench

Sit on a chair or bench with your legs extended in front of you, heels touching the floor. Grip the bench on both sides of your hips. Press through your palms to lift your hips and glutes off the bench. Slowly lower your bottom toward the floor by bending your arms at the elbows until you come to a ninety-degree angle. Your upper arms should be parallel to the floor or lower. Return to the top and squeeze your triceps without locking your elbows.

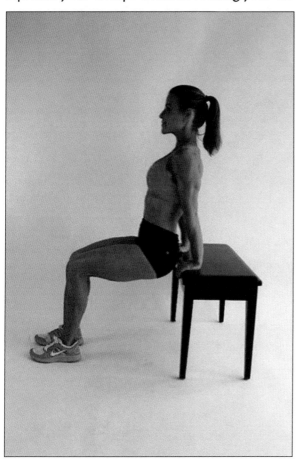
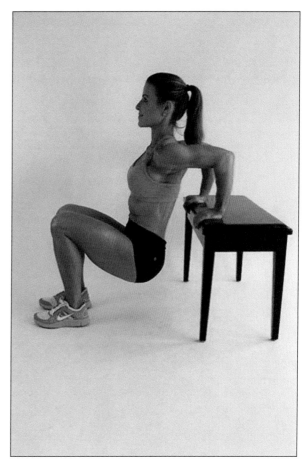

Russian Kicks

Sit down with your arms erect and your knees bent, fingers pointing toward your feet. Your legs are out in front of your body, glutes are off the floor, and your feet are facing forward. Engage your core as you start kicking your legs out in front, tapping the floor with your heels one leg at a time. Keep your arms straight and engage your triceps. Keep alternating for forty reps.

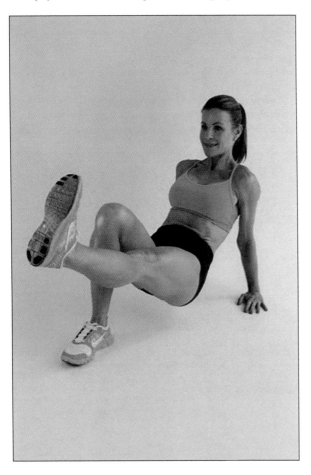
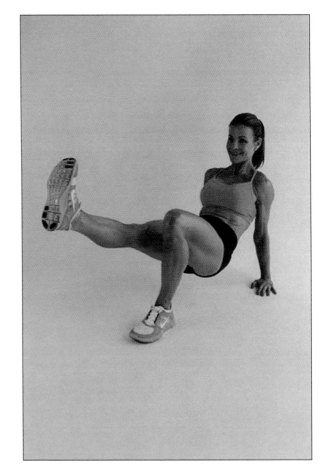

Cool Down and Stretch Out

Every workout session should be finished with *a cool down and stretching* period of about three to five minutes. It is very important to gradually bring your heart rate back down and to stretch out the muscles that you just worked so hard. Stretching prevents injury, speeds healing, and increases flexibility and overall joint mobility. As you do your stretches, make sure to challenge yourself to the point of slight discomfort, but never pain!

Always consume protein within thirty minutes of finishing your workout, as this is the optimal time frame for refueling your muscles to repair and rebuild them.

Chapter 21: Legs, Back, and Chest Workout

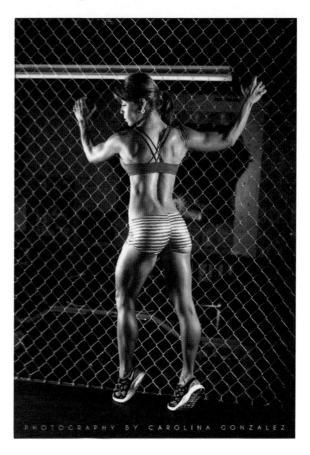

PHOTOGRAPHY BY CAROLINA GONZALEZ

This workout hits your glutes, legs, chest and back. It is a great workout that will get you lean and tight in all the right areas. As always, warm up and stretch out before you begin the weighted exercises. Also, remember your form and put your mind into your muscle to get the maximum benefit from each move. All you need is a workout mat and some dumbbells. This workout can be done anywhere.

Sumo Squats

Stand erect with your feet much wider than shoulder width apart. Toes should be pointing slightly out. Keep your head up, back arched, and chest up. Grab your dumbbells and with your body weight on your heels slowly lower yourself by bending your knees and pushing your glutes back. Lower until your thighs are parallel with the floor and your knees are at a ninety-degree angle. The deeper you squat, the more you engage your glutes! Pause and push back up to standing. As you get to the top of the move, squeeze your glutes hard. Repeat for reps.

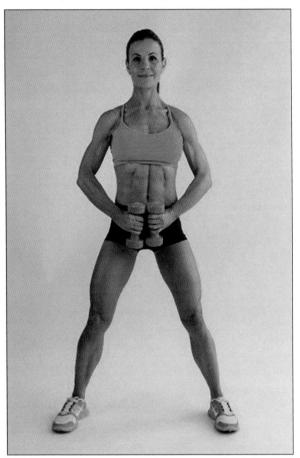 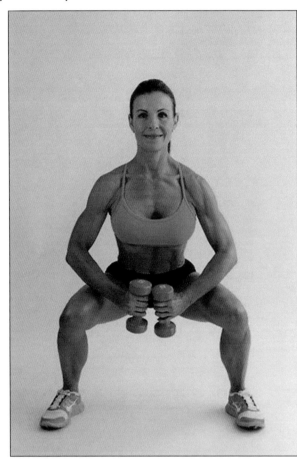

Perform thirty seconds of **jumping jacks** in between each set.

Dead Lifts

Stand erect with your feet shoulder width apart. Toes should be pointing straight forward and knees should be slightly bent. Keep your head up, back slightly arched, and chest elevated. Relax your arms down with dumbbells in hands, palms facing your thighs. Hinge at the hips while lowering your torso until it is parallel to the floor. You should maintain a slight back arch. Keep your chest up and shoulder blades contracted toward each other. The dumbbells should remain close to your legs throughout, as if you were shaving your legs. You should feel a good stretch in your hamstrings, and then you return up slowly while contracting hamstring and glutes. Come fully upright and push your hips forward, squeezing glutes hard at the top. Repeat for reps.

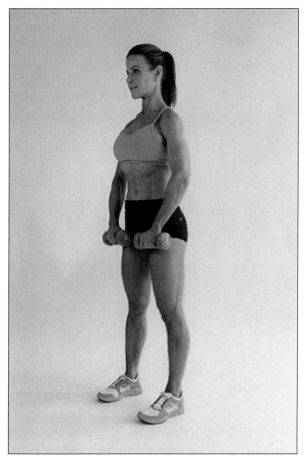 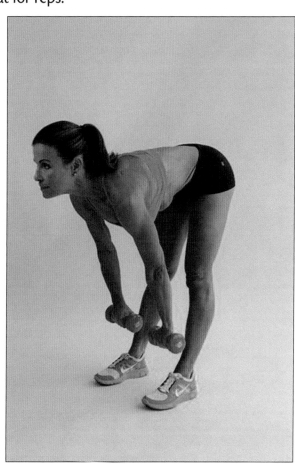

Perform thirty seconds of **high knees** in between sets.

Squats with Feet Together

Stand erect with your feet completely together. Toes should be pointing straight ahead. Keep your head up, back arched, and chest up. Grab your dumbbells and with your body weight on your heels slowly lower yourself by bending your knees and pushing your glutes back. Lower until your thighs are parallel with the floor and knees are at a ninety-degree angle. Pause and push back up to standing. As you get to the top of the move, squeeze your glutes hard. Repeat for reps.

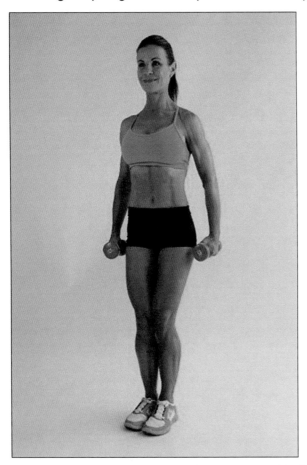 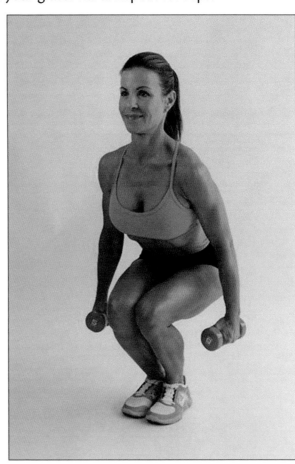

Perform thirty seconds of **mountain climbers** in between sets.

Weighted Plies, Feet Out

Stand erect with your feet wider than hip width apart and your toes pointed out. Keep your head up, back slightly arched, and chest elevated. Grasp a dumbbell with both hands and hold it in front of you. While keeping your torso as erect as possible, bend your hips and knees until your thighs are parallel to the floor. Squeeze your glutes and inner thighs, and while pushing through your heels, return to standing position. Do not lock your knees out, but continue squeezing your glutes. Repeat twenty times.

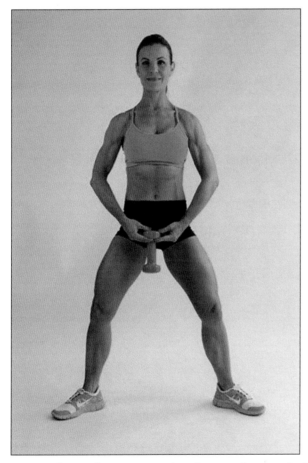 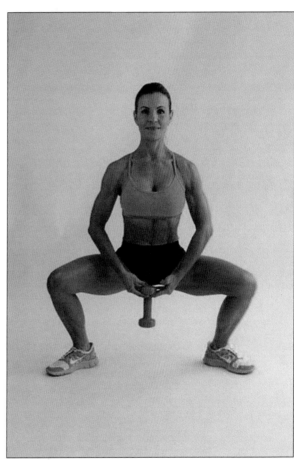

Perform thirty seconds of **squat jumps** in between sets.

Glute Bridge

Lie face up on the floor on a mat or towel. Arms are down by your sides. Bend your legs at ninety degrees, feet flat on the floor. Press through the heels and slowly lift your hips by contacting your glutes. Come all the way up and squeeze glutes hard while you hold for a count of two. Slowly return to starting position and repeat for thirty reps.

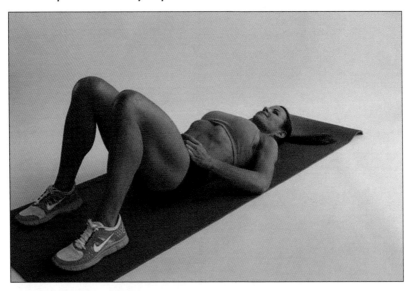

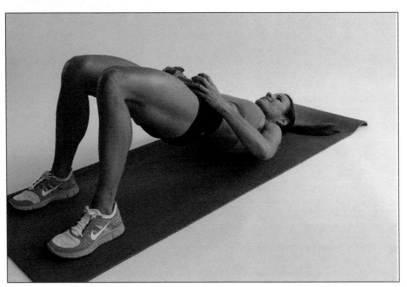

Perform thirty seconds of **jumping jacks in** between sets.

Standing Bent-Over Rows

Stand erect with your feet hip width apart and your toes pointed out. Bend at the waist. Keep your head up, back slightly arched, and chest elevated. Grasp a dumbbell in each hand and hold it in front of you with hands just inside shoulder width apart. Pull the weights up, while keeping them close to your body, leading with your elbows until your hands are just beneath your shoulders. Your elbows should be slightly higher than your wrists. Squeeze and slowly return to starting position. Repeat for reps.

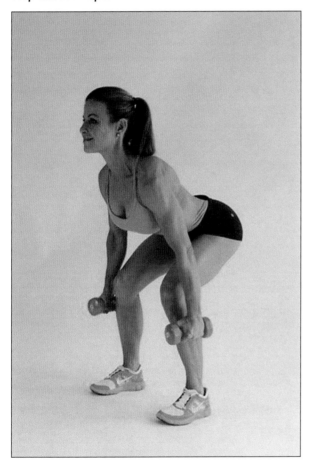 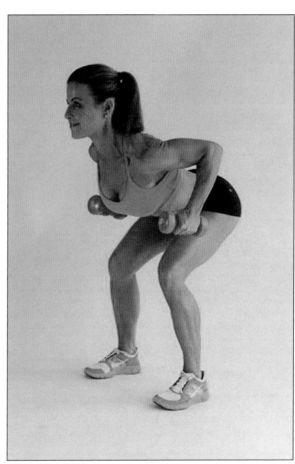

Perform thirty seconds of **high knees** in between sets.

Seated Rear Lateral Raise

Sit on a chair or stable surface. Your feet should be on the floor and your knees bent. Your torso is erect and your abs are engaged. Grab dumbbells and relax your arms by your sides, palms facing in. Slowly raise your arms up and out to the sides in a wide arc to about shoulder level, leading with your elbows. Slowly return to starting position. Repeat for reps.

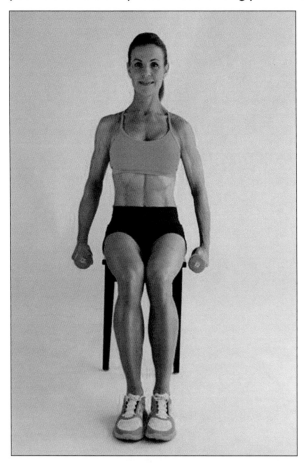 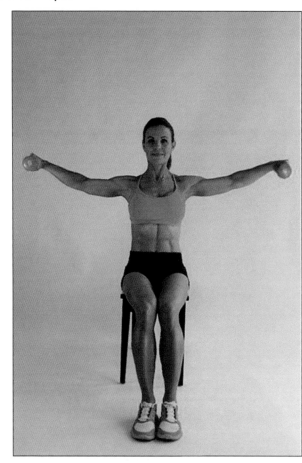

Perform thirty seconds of **jump rope** in between sets.

Chest Press on the Floor

Lie face up on the floor on a mat or towel. Arms are down by your sides. Bend your legs at ninety degrees, feet flat on the floor. Grab dumbbells in both hands, palms facing your feet and your elbows at ninety degrees. Tighten your core and glutes. Fully extend your arms in an arc up toward the ceiling. Control the movement so that dumbbells do not touch on top. Return by bringing your elbows to just parallel but still off the ground. Repeat for reps.

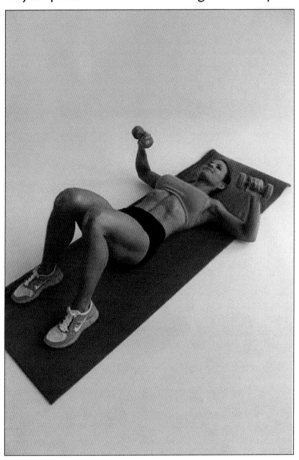 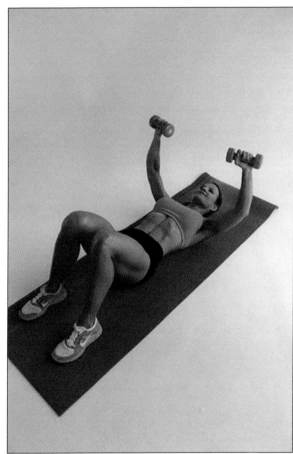

Push-ups

Get into push up position by making your body into a "plank." Your hands should be about four inches outside your shoulders. Contract your core, and keep your neck aligned with your spine. Keep your toes on the floor and your arms straight. Slowly lower your torso to the floor by opening your elbows out. When elbows form a ninety-degree angle and you are at the bottom, one inch off the floor, squeeze your pectorals, and then slowly return to start. Repeat for reps. (To make this exercise easier, start out by performing push-ups from a kneeling position, while tucking your hips down toward the floor.)

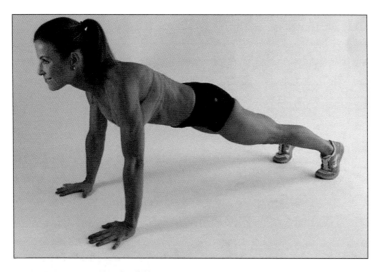

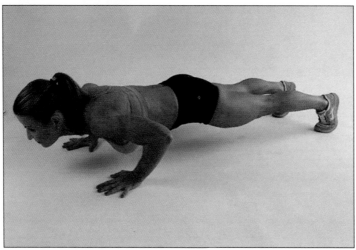

As always, cool down and stretch out. Enjoy your protein shake within thirty minutes of finishing your workout.

Chapter 22: Twenty-Minute Total-Body Fat Blaster

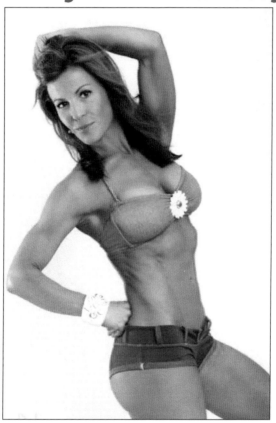

This workout can be done on days when you have less time and you want to rev up your metabolism with a super-efficient workout. Try to go for maximum exertion on each set and use the rest periods to bring down your heart rate slightly. This workout is like a HIIT session since you continuously spike your heart rate and then recover. It will elevate your metabolism and help you burn fat for the rest of the day.

Warm up by jogging in place for two minutes, and then stretch out.

Burpees: Three sets of twelve. Rest fifteen seconds between each set.

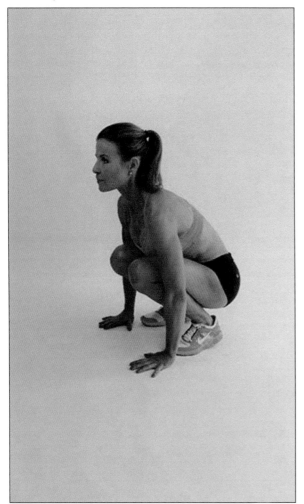

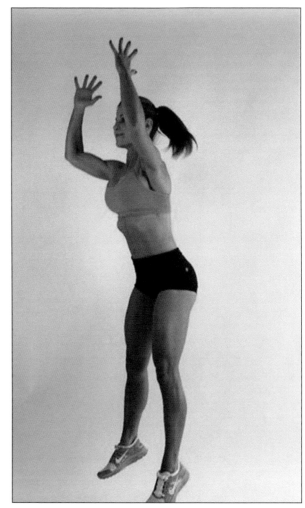

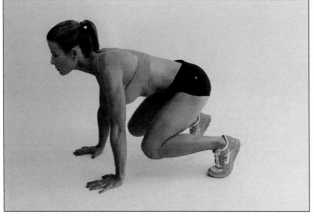

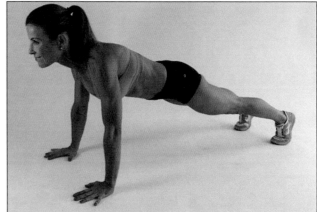

Jumping Jacks: Three sets of fifty. Rest fifteen seconds between each set.

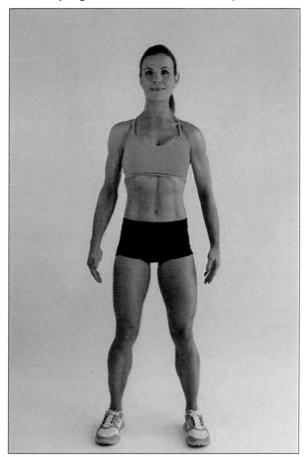
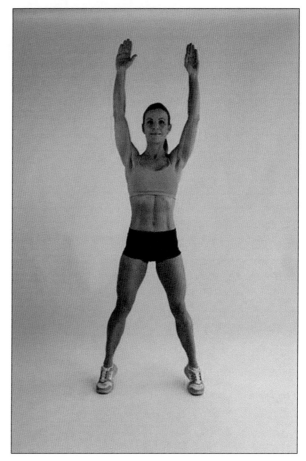

Body-Weight Squats with Kicks: Three sets of thirty. Rest fifteen seconds between each set.

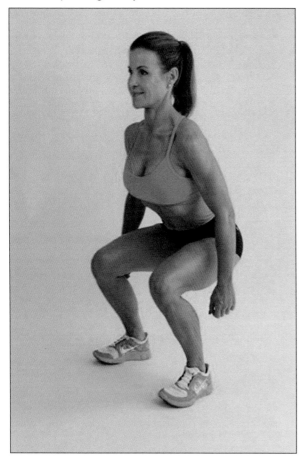 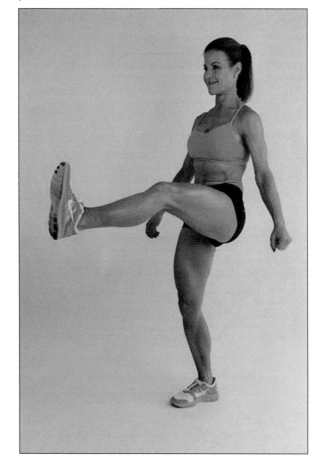

Mountain Climbers: Three sets of fifty. Rest fifteen seconds between each set.

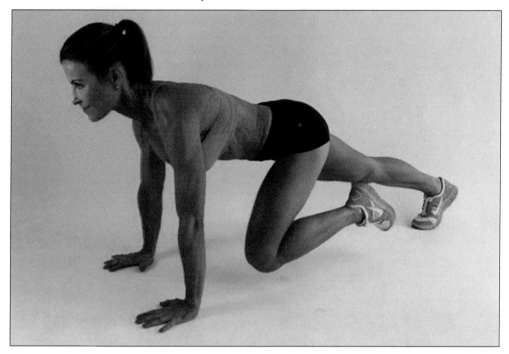

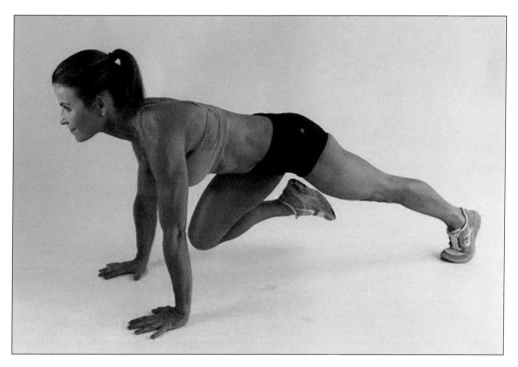

Step **O**ut, **A**lternating **L**unges: Three sets of thirty. Rest fifteen seconds between each set.

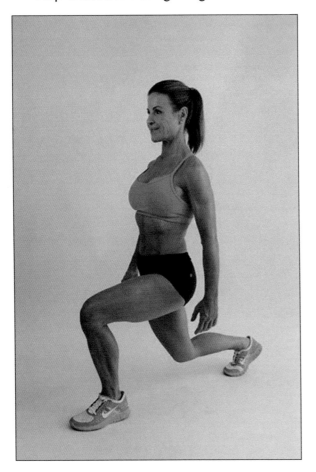 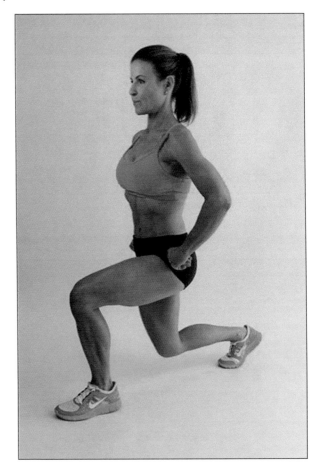

Split Squat Jumps: Three sets of twenty. Rest fifteen seconds between each set.

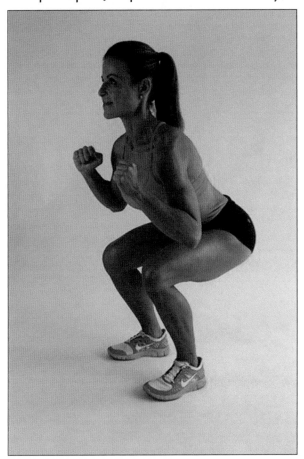 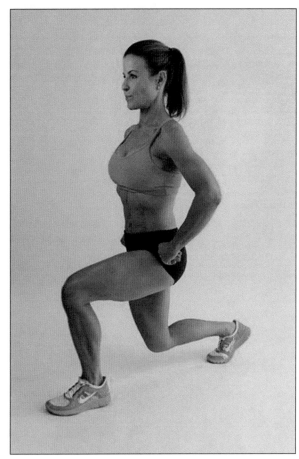

Push-ups: Three sets of twenty. Rest fifteen seconds between each set.

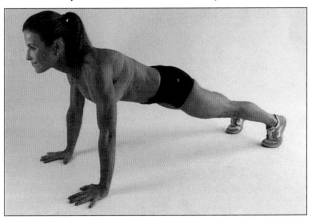 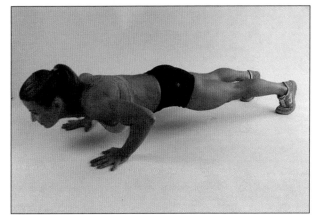

High Knees: Three sets of forty. Rest fifteen seconds between each set.

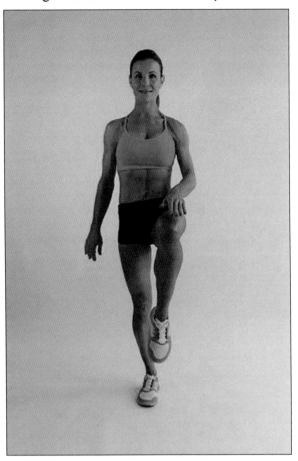 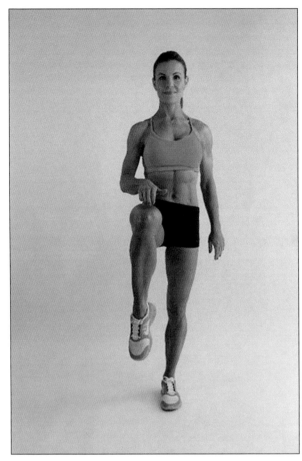

Cool Down and Stretch Out

Enjoy a protein shake made with one scoop of low-sugar hydrolyzed whey protein, glutamine, and water after your workout to enhance recovery and repair.

Final Words

You have started your journey to wonderful health and well-being. I congratulate you for your decision to take this important step. As you get more and more familiar with the eating program and the workouts, you will start to feel stronger, healthier, and leaner. Soon your new body will be your new "normal," and you will always strive to be in this state of great health and vitality. You will have more energy, greater focus, and feel younger and stronger than ever. It is important to stay at your new weight for at least three months, to avoid the weight creeping back on. To "reset" you new weight as your set point, maintain it by gradually increasing your caloric intake and by adopting my long term eating plan as your normal way of eating. You can add a cheat meal once a week, where you enjoy foods that are normally off limits, as long as you return to your new, Diet Diva Approved eating for the rest of the week.

I am also recommending that you look into the BodyFX products. They are simply the best supplements on the market today. All the products are sugar free, gluten free, NON GMO, free of artificial color or flavorings, and contain no additives or fillers. I use these products myself and love the results!

To find out more, simply visit: http://www.DietDivaBodyFX.com

Remember, you can always contact me directly for further personalized coaching or assistance.

I am here for *you*.

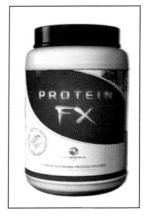

Unni Greene, The Diet Diva

www.UnniGreene.com

www.SoMiFitness.com

www.EatMoreToLoseMore.com

www.JanetTV.com

www.DietDivaBodyFX.com

www.jnlfusion.com

You Tube: www.youtube.com/somifitness305

Facebook: www.facebook.com/SoMiFitness

Pinterest: www.Pinterest.com/unnigreene

Twitter: www.twitter.com/somifitness

Instagram: www.instagram.com/unnigreene

Testimonials

I am a professional boxer. For most of my career, I boxed at 175 pounds. At the age of forty-three, an opportunity arose for me to box as a "super middleweight" at 168 pounds. I went to Unni and asked her if it would be possible for me to make that weight in less than eight weeks. She told me "yes, and you will never even be hungry." I was surprised, because I had always been hungry trying to make weight even at 175 pounds on my own. Unni was right. With her coaching me on my nutrition, I was able to make my weight at 168 pounds, and I was never hungry. But not only that, I was stronger than ever, and I was able to win my fight, knocking out my opponent, who was ten years younger than me! Unni knows what she is doing and is an essential part of my success at the age of forty-three.

Glen Johnson

Time **magazine "Boxer of the Year"**

World Middleweight Champion

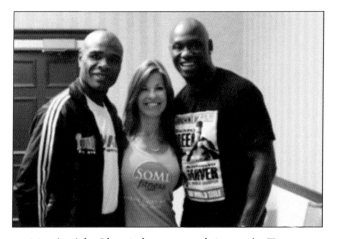

Unni with Glen Johnson and Antonio Tarver

I'd like to begin by thanking Unni, my trainer and nutritionist, who has become such an inspiration in my personal life. After all my hard work as a mother and a wife, I feel that I owe it to myself to make this new chapter of my life the best yet, living happier and healthier than ever. Unni's dedication, knowledge, and positive attitude are unmatched by any other nutrition expert or trainer I've ever known. Seeing her encourage me to take care of myself, and working with her as my personal trainer, has helped me to make positive changes in my eating habits; and working out harder with her has finally made it happen! At the age of forty, I can honestly say that thanks to Unni, I look and feel better than ever! With Unni's help and encouragement, I recently entered my first ever competition. I am proud to say that I took first place, and I have never felt better. Thank you, Unni!

Clara, wife, mother of two, forty years young!

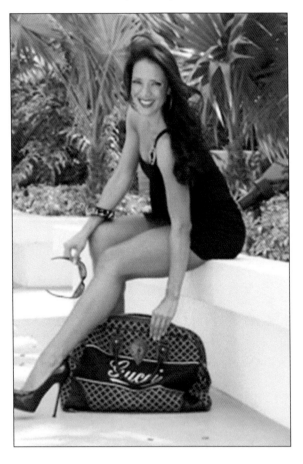

Being approximately eighty pounds overweight and severely obese, I knew I had to do something drastic. Having had prior knowledge of the expertise of Unni Greene, I knew that I had to go to her! So I enlisted another friend of mine, and off we went to Miami, where Unni is. We rented an apartment close to Unni's and Willie's gym with a workout room and pool, and we started out on our journey.

Unni met with me the following morning and designed a nutrition plan for me to follow, and so I did. I also attended her workout classes and tried as best I could to follow along with the other people in the class. Whenever I couldn't do something in the class (because I have two herniated discs in my back and one in my neck, which prevent me from doing many physical things), Unni would show me what I could do to still get the optimal results. The other people in the class were all great, too, and so supportive and positive to be around, which helped so much. The whole atmosphere was just wonderful!

I attended classes four to five days a week. In between classes, I rode the recumbent bike forty-five minutes a day! In six weeks, I lost twenty-eight pounds, and then I returned home. I have been continuing to exercise by going to a local gym and doing hot yoga. I now also have the JNL Fusion DVD program as well, I am still following Unni's "Eat More to Lose More" program, and I have lost forty-eight pounds so far! I don't know what I would have done without Unni. The program is phenomenal! Unni saved my life! Thanks again, Unni!

Paula, mother and wife, business owner

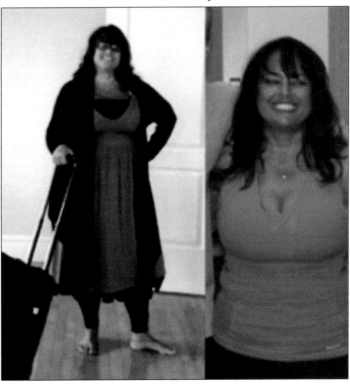

Unni, I want to thank you for helping me achieve the weight loss in eight weeks that I could not achieve by myself in four years. By following your meal plan I was never hungry, and I feel better than ever. Combined with your workouts, I look better than I did even before having kids! My husband is very happy, too! Thank you!

Luz, wife and mother of two

I wanted to thank you for helping me in my quest for health. My blood pressure is great, and I look to be off of medication soon. Also, since getting that kick-start with you, I have stayed involved in an exercise routine. You have made a huge difference in my life and, I am sure, in the lives of many others. I hope you never forget that you not only help people become healthier and live longer, but you also improve the *everyday* physical and emotional quality of their lives! I look forward to bending down to play with grandkids in years to come. Love you tons, and keep on keeping on!

Sonia, wife, mother of three, in her midforties

I started training with Unni back in December 2010, and although I had been working out before then for about thirteen years, her expertise in nutrition and training started changing

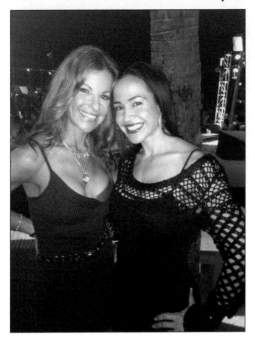

my body like never before. I am now thirty-six years old and a mother of two, and I have never felt better or been more toned and defined. Unni helped me lose body fat, gain lean, sexy muscles, and change my diet forever. When I met her, believe or not, I was a smoker, and as everyone knows most people have a fear that if they quit, they will gain weight. Well, thanks to Unni, I did not. With her encouragement and focus on health, I was able to stop smoking without gaining weight. In fact, her diet plan me lose fat and kept me at a healthy weight. Thanks to her intense workouts, the stress I thought I would release by smoking a cigarette was instead relieved by training with her. I have never felt better. Unni has helped me overcome many obstacles, and she is not only my mentor and inspiration, she is now a dear friend. Unni Greene is my Diet Queen. If you truly want to change your body forever and live a happy, healthy life no matter what your goals are, remember, it starts with a clean and healthy diet, and no one can show the way better than the Diet Diva.

Gysenia, wife, mother of two, business owner

Made in the USA
Lexington, KY
27 October 2014